PENGUIN BOOKS

HOW TO SURVIVE MEDICAL SCHOOL

Toni Martin is a graduate of Radcliffe College and the University of California at San Francisco Medical School. She lives in Oakland, California, with her husband, who is also a doctor, and their young son.

HOW TO SURVIVE MEDICAL SCHOOL

Toni Martin, M.D.

PENGUIN BOOKS

To my classmates

Penguin Books Ltd, Harmondsworth,
Middlesex, England
Penguin Books, 40 West 23rd Street,
New York, New York 10010, U.S.A.
Penguin Books Australia Ltd, Ringwood,
Victoria, Australia
Penguin Books Canada Limited, 2801 John Street,
Markham, Ontario, Canada L3R 1B4
Penguin Books (N.Z.) Ltd, 182–190 Wairau Road,
Auckland 10, New Zealand

First published in the United States of America by
Holt, Rinehart and Winston 1983
First published in Canada by
Holt, Rinehart and Winston of Canada, Limited, 1983
Published in Penguin Books 1984

LIBRARY OF CONGRESS CATALOGING IN PUBLICATION DATA
Martin, Toni.
How to survive medical school.
Includes index.
1. Medical education—Psychological aspects.
2. Medicine—Practice—Psychological aspects. 3. Medical
students—California—Biography. 4. Physicians—
California—Biography. I. Title.
[R737.M29 1984] 610'.7'1173 84-2856
ISBN 0 14 00.7319 1

Printed in the United States of America by
R. R. Donnelley & Sons Company, Harrisonburg, Virginia
Set in Sabon

Contents

Acknowledgments

When my brother-in-law decided to apply to medical school, he started asking questions that prompted me to think over my training. Despite his strong biology background and medical family, his concerns seemed much the same as my own seven years before. So I wrote this book to try to spare him and other medical students the trouble of reinventing the wheel. I hope he finds the book as useful as I found his questions.

My mother, who sent the first chapters to an agent when I was too pregnant to think, shares the credit for this book's publication with that agent, Jane Gelfman, and my editor Bobbi Mark. Their faith kept me writing when new motherhood threatened to overwhelm me.

Several friends lent me typewriters and a quiet place when the newborn left no peace at home. My neighbor Karen Roselle typed most of the manuscript and helped me see my words from the point of view of an intelligent nonmedical reader.

Finally, whatever perspective I was able to bring to the subject I owe to my husband and son, whose constant love keeps me from taking the world too seriously.

Introduction

This little book is about what happens to some of the loneliest people on earth: medical students and premedical students. Burdened by the fabulous expectations of their parents and incessant scholastic demands, they must negotiate a competitive course toward a goal they can scarcely envision. Their egos are routinely shattered by everyone from the secretaries at the admissions office to the professor on rounds. It happens to practically everyone, but since their classmates are all pretending to be breezing through there is little commiseration. Once home, they are expected to make up for their forced absence with lighthearted banter and passionate sex, even if they have been awake thirty-six hours watching a patient die. Their former friends accuse them of being rich doctors, when in fact their income qualifies them for food stamps. Through it all, they are reminded how lucky they are to have made it to medical school.

While I believe that loneliness is an equal-opportunity emotion, the more nontraditional the student, the less support is forthcoming. Talking with the women in my class, I discovered that the family of one Jewish woman had greeted her decision to enter medical school by reciting the prayer for the dead, an Indian woman had broken an arranged engagement, and a Chinese woman was temporarily estranged from her family. My father merely asked, "Why do you want to deal with the shit of the world?"—which in retrospect seems a reasonable question. "Ah, yes," they always smile and say, "but you'd do it again, wouldn't you?" I honestly don't know. What I do know is that my years of medical training were not the happiest ones of my life. Anyone who tells you different is probably independently wealthy and went to medical school before 1960.

But with the help of this book, anyone, even a black woman like me—with two strikes against her—can get through medical school. Just remember: My smiling theme song could have been "I Did It Their Way," but my motto was "Don't Let the Bastards Get You Down."

HOW TO
SURVIVE
MEDICAL
SCHOOL

1

THE
APPLICATION

TO BE A DOCTOR

Hypnotize a hundred first-year medical students, and you will hear a hundred different reasons why an otherwise rational, reasonably bright individual would want to be a doctor. Some yielded to parental pressure, some wanted to be rich, some wanted to save the world, some wanted to save themselves. One may have had an ailing parent, another was hospitalized after an automobile accident. There will be a medic and a nutritionist alongside an engineer and a missionary. For every student who idolizes Albert Schweitzer and Linus Pauling, there will be one inspired by Ché Guevara or William Carlos Williams. I first remember thinking seriously about a medical career in high school, after reading *The Plague* by Albert Camus, but I had classmates who declared a subspecialty in their elementary school yearbooks and consequently never heard of Camus.

The only common chord in this symphony of aspirations is, with rare exception, blithe ignorance of what physicians actually do, or more accurately, the boundaries of the physician's role in today's society. Seven years into his surgical training, the entrepreneur may well wish that he had opted for an M.B.A. At the same time, the crusader may have realized that his patients see him as an obstacle in their quest for self-destruction. The mild-mannered academic will learn to play hardball with the boys in the department or resign himself to obscurity. Fortunately, medical school provides at least four years of soul-consuming toil to keep your mind off your dreams. After medical school, the enterprising student can, with no difficulty, stay in training for at least five years—ten if he chooses a surgical subspecialty. By the time such a physician actually practices, he or she is lucky to remember the kid who started anatomy, much less that kid's dreams.

So don't worry if the best reason you can articulate for applying to medical school is that you like science and you like people. It is the gut feeling that hit you at age five or age thirty that will sustain you when the dollar bill and the revolution fail. Only when that is lacking would I counsel another course, but you wouldn't listen, anyway.

WHAT LIES AHEAD

Before I launch into a description of the application process, let me outline the stages of medical training. After college comes medical school, traditionally four years, although very few schools shorten it to three. There are also rare combined college-medical school programs requiring only six years of unimaginable intensity, but that is an option only for those still in high school. After medical school comes a year of internship, now sometimes called the first year of residency. In the old days, internship was the first exposure to hands-on patient care, but now the last two years of medical school are also spent in the hospital, so the transition is not quite as violent. Nevertheless, a year of internship is currently required for licensure in thirty-five of the fifty states so it is still part of the making of the doctor.

A formal written exam is required before a license to practice is granted. In Texas, Louisiana, and the Virgin Islands, the Federation Licensing Exam (FLEX), an all-inclusive preclinical and clinical test, is the only exam recognized. Most states recognize either the FLEX or the National Medical Board exams, a series of three tests taken at the end of the second and fourth years of medical school and at the end of the internship. The first test deals with basic sciences or preclinical work, the second with the clinical work of medical school, and the third with patient management.

After the U.S.-trained physician is certified by one of these exams (foreign medical graduates follow a different route), he or she is free to hang out a shingle and call him or herself a general practitioner. However, few physicians exercise this option nowadays; most continue for further training called residency. The terms *intern* and *resident*, by the way, are holdovers from the days when doctors in training were required to live in the hospital, received no pay, and were not allowed to marry. If you make it to medical school, you will hear quite a bit about this golden age of medicine from professors complaining about how soft students have it today.

Residencies vary in length, depending on the specialty. Surgeons train the longest, with general surgery requiring five to six years after medical school, urology and orthopedics four to five, cardiac or neurosurgery about seven. The total time of internship and residency varies from program to program. Obstetricians complete a three-year residency after internship for a total of four years. We primary-care physicians finish first; pediatricians, internists, and family practitioners do one year of internship and two years of residency. So do anesthesiologists and dermatologists.

At the end of residency programs, the now graying physicians face more board examinations for certification in their fields. These exams are not required to practice, however. A doctor can finish just two years of general surgery and call himself a surgeon if a hospital will give him privileges. Board certification is a crude method of quality assurance and confers prestige.

Finally, after residency, the physician may choose to pursue subspecialty training as a fellow. For instance, in internal medicine, I had a choice of fellowships in pulmonary medicine, gastroenterology, and cardiology, to name a few. An orthopedic surgeon may pursue a hand surgery fellowship or a sports medicine fellowship. A confusing aspect of this nomenclature is that the title "fellow" does not indicate how many years of postgraduate training a physician has completed. At the end of a two-year neonatology fellowship, a pediatrician will have spent fewer years in training than his friend the sixth-year cardiac surgery resident. There is also another category of doctor in training skulking the wards: the chief resident. In medicine and pediatrics, the chief resident is chosen by the faculty to fulfill an administrative and teaching role as a sort of junior, junior faculty member. The chief residency is an extra year of training. In the surgical world, the chief has the same role but performs his duties in his last year of training, in rotation with the others in his year. Actually, some medical chief residencies rotate also, but this is the exception, not the rule.

Another confusing aspect of medical training is that applications and preparations for the next phase always begin earlier than the casual observer would expect. The application for medical school should be completed during the summer after junior year of college. Scheduling of clinical work for the third and fourth years of medical school must be largely completed second year. Applications for internship should be started by the end of third year and completed early in the fourth. Some very popular residencies such as psychiatry, dermatology, and ophthalmology accept applicants three years before the starting date.

In the organization of this book, I have tried to ease the dilemma of the medical student coping with the exigencies of now while planning for the day after tomorrow by including some information pertinent to the next endeavor in each year's chapter. For example, the chapter on second year discusses how to order clinical rotations in the following year. My goal is not to jump the gun, but to keep the medical student from scrambling to catch up.

PRE-MED COURSES

Pre-med courses are the first of a series of institutionalized hurdles designed to weed out the mellow student. They are not entirely successful only because geniuses and schizophrenics can be mellow and compulsive at the same time. The rest of us find ourselves more and more punctilious as our medical education progresses. I therefore disagree with the wide body of opinion that holds that pre-med courses are useless. The content may slip from the synapses, but the process remains. And a doctor should be careful in checking orders, checking tests, and checking people. Now, I don't think organic chemistry is the only course capable of teaching meticulous study habits. Intensive Urdu would serve the same purpose if medical schools cared about it. Perhaps they should agree on a different course every ten years or so, if only to spare the organic chemists the teaching burden.

Organic chemistry, incidentally, will probably be the first course the pre-med student will take in which the instructors just won't seem to like him. It will not be the last. The reason is that the chemists resent having to teach students who for the most part have no interest in the subject apart from their final grades. Since medicine is an applied science, instructors in all the so-called basic sciences, such as anatomy, physiology, and histology are prone to the same point of view. They see medical students as boorish and greedy. Since the pre-med and medical students resent the requirements, which they perceive as irrelevant, mutual scorn and lack of interest are the order of the day. For those of us whose impetus to perform involves seeking the approval of an instructor (a particularly nefarious but common product of early female socialization), this scorn can be devastating. Somehow the well-accepted dictum that students tend to perform in accordance with their teachers' expectations has not filtered up to science professors. So teachers often sarcastically dismiss the class as "only pre-meds" barely capable of parroting predigested summaries.

Of course, the sheer quantity of material that the pre-med or medical student must tackle, if not learn, works against both student and professor. I remember a friend warning me that I would flunk out if I persisted in actually trying to read the pathology textbook with the pretty pictures rather than memorize the lecture summaries. She was right, too. Fortunately, most medical texts are so tedious that the temptation does not often arise.

I served as a student member of the admissions committee at my medical school for two years, so I know that it is important to do well in pre-med courses. They are evaluated separately from your overall grade-point average and your science grade point. On the other hand, if you botch a course, or if you fulfilled the requirements years ago when you thought you were going to be a concert pianist, it is definitely worth your while to take some other science courses and do well. Remember that, by and large, no one will know the course description, so don't volunteer that Biology 298 was an ecology course that involved four field trips and a paper—just record the A. If you really have been out of school awhile, better take something more serious, as much to test your stamina as to impress the medical school. If you have only taken one biology course in ten years, you are more likely to be asked about it, too.

As long as you do well in the pre-med courses, there is no reason to force yourself to major in biology or chemistry if that is not your inclination. College is your last chance at a general education, so take advantage of it. Medical schools will not penalize you for it. Oh, you might have to do some fancy talking about the relationship of Nordic myth to medicine, but just think about it before your interview and you'll come up with something. If the pre-meds who don't enjoy chemistry leave that field as much as possible to those who do, everyone will be happier. The pre-med who takes anatomy to get a head start on medical school becomes the medical student who takes the coronary care unit elective to get a head start on internship and the resident who takes cardiology to get a head start on fellowship. Sure, he looks bright for the first week or so of each new stage, but he's cheated himself out of any enjoyment of the present or the future, since he's impatient in the one and bored in the other.

Pre-med and medical students are too accomplished at postponing gratification. By assuming that nothing counts until the M.D. degree, they lose years of their lives. Remember, college, medical school, and postgraduate training can take ten to fifteen years. If you don't stop to smell the flowers when you can, you will regret, or worse, resent it later. Believe me, the world doesn't need any more bitter doctors.

Finally, if you have an opportunity, take a Spanish course. There are not many training centers left that do not serve a Spanish-speaking population, and even a little pidgin Spanish goes a long way. In another sort of world, medical schools in California and New York would require a year of Spanish; it has certainly been as useful to me as physics.

THE MEDICAL COLLEGE ADMISSIONS TEST

Anyone on the brink of applying to medical school should realize by now that anytime someone tells you that there is no point in studying for a test because it measures only aptitude or the scope is too broad, you'd better hit the books. Study by yourself or take a course; it will help. Take the Medical College Admissions Test (MCAT) the academic year before you apply (in the spring of your junior year rather than the fall of your senior year) because your file will not be complete until those scores are in. Repeat the test only if you have reason to believe that you will do substantially better, since the latest scores will delay your application. Here again, the admissions committee is largely concerned with your science score. Tell your mother how well you did on the rest.

THE APPLICATION

For some reason, students who have otherwise calculated every move from kindergarten to fellowship sometimes slip up when it comes to the application. I don't mean that the typing is lousy, although it won't hurt to have it look spiffy. I mean they leave out crucial information, which delays processing, or they leave out the essay, which at my medical school could cost them an interview, since the essay was assigned points in screening just like the grade point or the letters of recommendation. The essay is the only part of the application that you can influence significantly, so write a good one. Don't send a poem; it will set you apart, but it will take more time to evaluate and will exasperate the screener. If you can't spell, have someone proofread your piece. Contrary to popular opinion, most doctors are marginally literate and are offended by gross grammatical errors. Don't make your essay too long, but even the best-chosen sentence will not suffice.

Don't try to be too original. You are expected to write about why you want to be a doctor, so make a stab at it. If you have spent the last ten years gathering manioc in Brazil, give the screener a hint why. If your mother is a doctor and truly influenced your decision to apply, say so, but don't spend the whole essay extolling her virtues. If you are a born-again Christian and feel you must cite God as your inspiration, just remember the person reading your essay probably isn't and will appreciate some less spiritual discussion as well. In general, address your thoughts to a sympathetic young doctor (older doctors are smart enough to avoid admissions committees) who wants to know what makes you tick, not the details of your research on squid axons. If you know a doctor who would be willing to criticize your essay, preferably someone who is or has been involved in the admissions process, by all means take advantage of the opportunity.

EXTRACURRICULAR ACTIVITIES

In this day of grade inflation and intense competition, when medical schools are forced to choose among hundreds of students with straight A averages, extracurricular activities have assumed an importance that I think is perfectly ridiculous. I don't see why participation in the Stanford marching band should have any bearing on acceptance to medical school, but that is the way the game is played; so the complete pre-med should wrack his brain for the most impressive way to list his leisure pursuits. I always had difficulty with this because I am not a joiner, and the hobbies I actually have—reading, writing, knitting, cooking, hiking—would look better on an application for a senior citizens' home than one for medical school.

Try to list a sport; doctors like jocks. "Tennis team" looks a lot better than "tennis," but "intramural football" looks okay. Running is fine, but list your weekly mileage. If you are a marathoner, so much the better. Many physicians run; it's a good way to burn up all that excess self-discipline. Whatever you do, describe it in as much detail as space allows. They are looking for evidence that you actually pursued an activity with some regularity and commitment.

Any pre-med organizations count, but not much. A smidgen of research and a volunteer job working with people, preferably in a medical setting, are almost de rigueur. Both can be quite valuable experiences, worthy of undertaking in and of themselves, but all too often they look more impressive on paper than in real life. You will be asked about your activities in your interviews, so don't make them up. I've known an interviewer to check for calluses on learning that a student played the acoustic bass.

Again, realize you are not alone. Very few pre-med students are in a position to make a meaningful contribution to the health care system. Your pre-med experiences should expose you to patients and lab rats, not launch your career. Don't spend three summers as an orderly unless you really want to; there's no upward mobility. Above all, don't use the space for the essay to finish listing your activities. Write an essay and add an extra sheet of paper to itemize your scientific publications.

LETTERS OF RECOMMENDATION

This is another area of the application process where students can unwittingly fall short of the mark. The fault generally lies with halfhearted recommendations or inappropriate choices for references. Ideally, letters should come from full professors in the sciences who know you well and will praise you as the finest candidate for medical school they have seen in the last forty years. Obviously, this is not easy to arrange. You must cultivate references from early on in your college career. Go to meet professors during their office hours and give them a chance to associate you with your name. Do well in their courses. Arrange for an independent study with someone you genuinely admire, and work like the devil. If you are far from your undergraduate years, do the best you can; you may want to consider taking another science course just for the recommendation. Don't pester your professors, though. They are wise to your strategy and skeptical of constant attention. A summer job involving research is another excellent way of securing a recommendation.

Once you have picked your professors, ask them point-blank whether they feel capable of writing you a strong recommendation. You may regard a professor as your personal guru while he or she sees you as Whatshisname in the second row. Remember, professors have many students, and especially if your standing in the class is not high, you may not be among the chosen in their eyes. The reference you choose must know you well enough to write about you as a person, apart from your letter grade. On the other hand, a personal friend of the family, even an M.D., is not a good reference unless he or she can judge your performance in an intellectual pursuit, not just attest to your impeccable genes. It is important to know the quality of a reference at the outset, before the letter has been written. Many schools nowadays have pre-medical committees that screen recommendations, editing them so that they read like the blurbs on book jackets. This is an immense service to the applicant, who in the past might have learned of a tepid letter only at the time of an interview. In fact, if your school does not have such a committee, make every attempt to read the letters yourself, or designate your adviser as official screener. One reason schools such as Harvard have such impressive acceptance figures for their pre-med students is that a Harvard pre-med committee letter could make Attila the Hun look like a promising candidate.

Since it is advantageous to apply early, keep on top of the progress of your recommendations. If someone is late in writing, remind him or her obsequiously but at reasonably frequent intervals. Along this line, if the Nobel Prize–winner in the department has supervised you in the lab for the last three years but will be abroad on sabbatical during your senior year, make sure his letter is in your file before he boards the plane to Paris.

Finally, if you are still at the stage of declaring your major, think of the problem of references before you sign up for your school's most crowded major. My undergraduate area of concentration was geology, where the ratio of full professors to undergraduate concentrators was one to one. I never considered medical school when I made that choice, but it was much easier for me than for my friends in biology to rustle up someone important who knew me when the time came.

THE INTERVIEW

Everyone will tell you that the interview is important, if not crucial. And they are quite right. If you are denied an interview at the school of your choice and you believe your record is competitive, appeal the decision and ask for a review of your record. At best, this strategy will earn you an interview; at worst, you will gain some insight into why the interview was refused, which will help you improve your application for the next year. But be realistic. If your grade-point average is 2.4, you already know why you weren't chosen for an interview.

Once the interview is scheduled, take a moment to congratulate yourself. You have already managed to distinguish yourself from the hordes at the gate. Now you must give the medical school a reason to select you from among the hundreds of students interviewed.

Interviewing skills are the subjects of books in their own right; here I can only touch on a few of the principles. First, in order to make a good impression, you should dress like a professional, even if all your friends in medical school wear jeans. Most of the other applicants, male and female, will be wearing suits, and this is one time that you would rather not be distinguished from the crowd. Your goal should be to dress so that the interviewer will think not about your attire, but about you.

Next, try to anticipate what the interviewer is going to ask. If you have no idea, ask some of your friends who were interviewed recently. The basic questions don't change much from year to year: "Why did you decide to go into medicine?" and all its variations. You will probably be asked about your major, particularly if it is not a traditional pre-med major; your extracurricular activities; any time off between undergraduate work and applying to medical school. You may be asked to comment on an important issue within medicine or to identify the most pressing problem facing society. You may be asked about family, your spouse's plans, your hometown. You will almost certainly be asked, "What do you see yourself doing in ten years?"

All of these are difficult questions that require forethought. Interviewers are not supposed to ask sexist questions such as "What would you do if you became pregnant?" But if you want to get into that school, how much you complain is a matter for your own conscience. Questions such as "Have you considered how medical school will affect your family life?" are probably legitimate as long as they are routinely addressed to applicants of both sexes, which, of course, is impossible for any single applicant to ascertain. The stress interview is supposed to be passé, but one recent applicant I know faced "Well, if you gave up painting, why won't you give up medicine?" Another had to fend off "You think you're pretty smart, don't you?"

I think the ideal way to prepare is to have a medical student you know role-play an interview with you, full of slippery questions based on your background. Remember that at some schools the interviewer will not have access to your folder, so you'll have to explain your existence from scratch, while at others he or she will have studied your record and will ask you to explain away every B on it or will edit your essay. At times like these, it is crucial to remain calm and bite your tongue. If the interviewer wanders off on a tangent and you haven't had a chance to touch on an aspect of your application that you regard as essential, do try to nudge him or her in your direction before it's too late. Just because your schedule reads "Interview 10:00 to 11:00 A.M." doesn't mean you'll have the whole hour. Often, busy physicians are unavoidably late or have a lecture scheduled for the same time as the second half of your interview.

Which brings to mind another important point—you must shine from the opening salvo. If you are shy and warm to people slowly, try to practice making a stronger initial impression. I can't count the number of times I have thought students showed promise toward the end of the interview when they finally began to relax, but it was too late to talk more. The conscientious interviewer tries to take nervousness into account, but a student who answers in monosyllables for the first half-hour is always going to be at a disadvantage. On the other hand, don't pour out your heart to anyone, no matter how sympathetic that person seems to be. Be particularly wary of this with student interviewers. If you wouldn't tell a faculty member you actually flunked biochem once, don't tell a student.

Be prepared to ask a few questions of your own. This is easy when your interview is first on the agenda but may be forced if you've already had two student tours. Just ask the same questions again, if necessary. Ask about the school's strength in research or clinical areas, about teaching hospitals, about the demographics of recent classes. A faculty member probably won't know much about student housing or percentage of elective time in the fourth year, so save those questions for students. I was always curious to learn what sort of M.D. my interviewer was, so I generally asked, but I'm not sure that's standard practice.

Finally, remember that your interviewer was undoubtedly not trained to talk to pre-med students. She may be new to the admissions committee. He may not have spoken to anyone more assertive than his research animals in years. In other words, they have problems, too. As a student interviewer, I was often so depressed that I found it difficult to believe anyone could want to apply to medical school, even though I was only two years removed from the experience myself. So don't feel your interview was a failure because you did not sense any overt positive emotion and the conversation was halting. I remember some animated discussions with glib students whom I ultimately ranked rather low.

ACCEPTANCE AND REJECTION

The interview is a microcosm of the entire admissions procedure: inefficient and arbitrary. A lottery would be just as fair, but is philosophically distasteful. So do your best, but brace yourself for startling inconsistencies. All is not fair. On the other hand, a good student should be accepted somewhere, even if it's not his first-choice school. If you sent out ten applications (a standard number), including an application to your state school, and you were rejected without an interview by all of them, you need to sit down and do some soul-searching. First, I would again suggest contacting the schools in an effort to learn what part of your application was deficient. If they can identify one area that was not satisfactory and indicate that the rest was acceptable, you can buckle down and study for the MCAT again, or try to pull up your science average with a few more courses. In other words, you have a fair prospect of strengthening your application enough by the following year to make it worthwhile to reapply. If they thought your whole record was weak, however, you face a more difficult decision. Simply resubmitting the same weak application year after year does not improve your chances. Persistence alone will not impress the committee. You need to change your application substantially to improve your ranking—a change that may require years and thousands of dollars to achieve.

To many students, any investment is worthwhile if it means a place in medical school. They repeat all their pre-med courses and their MCATs and apply three or four times if necessary. Others opt for a foreign medical school at this point. I would be the last to counsel giving up. I will emphasize, however, that after the third application, the admissions committees have your number and your prospects are vanishingly slim. At least consider allied health fields, nursing and nurse practitioner programs, physician's assistant programs, physical therapy, respiratory therapy, medical engineering, clinical pharmacology. I do not mention doctoral programs only because they tend to be even more rigorous than medical school.

If you are reapplying and have time to kill, consider a

master's degree in a health-related field. A master's in public health is a requirement today for some physician jobs in the public arena, and it certainly won't hurt your application to do well in such a program. If you have the money, travel some or, better yet, work in a clinic or hospital abroad. Some candidates fail their interviews because they seem to have no interests beyond home and school. Travel gives you something to talk about and demonstrates initiative and maturity.

On to those who made the interview but were still not accepted. If you fall into this category, you can assume you already have a solid application. Gild it, following the advice above. Work particularly on how you present yourself during the interview itself, for that was almost certainly your Waterloo.

Finally, a few words about a more pleasant dilemma: choosing between multiple acceptances. To win at this game, you must always hold a place somewhere, but never more than one. Send in the deposit to your last-choice school even if you are accepted in August of your senior year and you are almost certain you'll hear from schools higher on your list. As my pre-med adviser put it, "A hundred dollars is cheap for a place in medical school." As soon as you hear from a school higher on your list, however, release that place to someone else. It is unconscionable to hold several places at once, given the competition to get in at all. Besides, you won't get away with it, because there is a centralized computer to which the schools report their acceptances in order to keep track of who is going where.

While you are trying to make up your mind, visit the schools, talk to the students. All medical students are depressed, but some are more depressed than others. If you are interested in clinical medicine, ask about teaching hospital affiliations. Third- and fourth-year students can tell you if they are tripping over each other on the wards for lack of patients. Ask about elective time, especially in the clinical years. Ask about testing. We had an exam every time we turned around, but at least one school I visited relied on self-evaluation until the first part of the National Board second year. The curricula don't vary much, but some schools teach by organ system instead of discipline, that is, anatomy, physiology, histology of the lung, then of the heart, rather than anatomy of the body, physiology of the body, histology of the body. If you are applying with a spouse, consider the size of the school carefully. My husband and I were attracted to a school with sixty students and 10 percent black enrollment until we realized that we would be one-third of the black students in the entering class.

Location and cost are essential considerations. Since you will have to apply for internships later, wherever you settle now need not be permanent but you can expect cultural differences. An Eastern friend who chose Brigham Young University Medical School recalls his first surface anatomy class with chagrin. When a fellow student volunteered to take off his shirt so that the instructor could demonstrate the muscles of the chest, my friend started joking about the student's unseasonably heavy undergarment. He stopped quickly when he realized no one else was laughing. In fact, almost everyone in the room was wearing the same garment, as do most adult Mormons. He spent the next four years trying to pry his foot out of his mouth.

Ten years ago, when I applied, I was counseled not to consider money as a factor in my choice of school. My premed adviser thought I was crazy to turn down a prestigious private school in favor of a good state school. But I just didn't believe that it "wouldn't make any difference" if my husband and I, both starting medical school, accumulated $40,000 in debts, as opposed to less than $20,000. Maybe it wouldn't have mattered if our families were wealthy. But choosing the state school was the smartest move we ever made. As it is we feel that we are in hock to Uncle Sam for life because of educational loans. It is not true that you can pay them back immediately out of astronomical earnings. It will be even less true if doctors' incomes fall with the predicted glut. Don't choose a school you would not otherwise consider because it is cheap, but do check the bottom line if the schools are comparable.

If you've never been west of Manhattan and you're alone, medical school may not be the time to get to know Seattle. Just because you're grown up doesn't mean you can't get homesick. Aim for a school where you'll feel comfortable, not like a pioneer.

BEFORE SCHOOL STARTS

In general, I would recommend spending the summer before medical school as idly as possible, since there's plenty of work around the corner. But if you're champing at the bit and summer anatomy is offered, go ahead and take it. Tackling that course alone will defuse anxiety and lighten your load the rest of the year. Financial realities being what they are, however, most students will have to work. That's fine, but allow at least a few weeks to install yourself in your new life. It is bad form to skip the first lab to be home when the furniture arrives. Whatever you end up doing, don't worry about everyone else. You'll be as ready as your classmates.

2

FIRST YEAR: HITTING THE BOOKS

Anatomy dominates the first year of medical school. Much of the anxiety of starting school focuses on that course, partly because of the mystique surrounding cadavers, partly because fewer undergraduates have been exposed to anatomy than to biochemistry or microbiology. At most schools, dissections are performed by groups of students because, mercifully, the supply of dead bodies is limited. So anatomy becomes the social focus of the first year, with dissection partners constituting, for better or for worse, your closest peer group. Anatomy is also a humbling course for whiz kids with intuitive analytical skills or photographic memories, since an anatomy practical does not provide problems to solve and since memory without a sense of spatial relationships serves as well as chopsticks with a steak.

For most students, particularly those who were humanities concentrators, anatomy is the first test of medical school macho. "Are you tough enough?" was the metaquestion posed by the interviewers last year. Now, finally starting after years of anticipation, the question has been internalized. "Am I tough enough?" reads each student's face as she or he struggles to concentrate on the lecture before the first lab. That lecture was forbidding rather than welcoming: warnings about the sanctity of the human body and a brief history of medical grave robbers over the centuries. At that point, I remember agreeing with the lecturer that it was fortunate that cadavers were provided for us, but secretly acknowledging to myself that if obtaining cadavers illegally were still part of the curriculum I would have sought another line of work.

The next lecture covered the details of dissecting the breast. I suppose the breasts were a logical place to start, but we women shrank from this initial approach. So did the men when many weeks later we reached the scrotum. After two introductory lectures, I felt more anxious than I had when I arrived, which I hardly would have thought possible.

I remember entering the dissecting laboratory and reeling from the smell of formalin. I remember one woman in my group of four crying, "Oh, it looks just like my mother before she died!" when she saw our cancer-ridden emaciated corpse. And I remember refusing to name the cadaver Gertrude since that is my mother's name. But I don't recall who made the first cut or how we managed for the next few hours. We just did it, that's all.

Again, anatomy is symbolic of the medical school process. Day after day, particularly in the clinical years, medical students are called upon to perform tasks for which they feel neither psychologically nor intellectually prepared. "See one, do one, teach one," a motto that is constantly repeated, is really a creed allowing for no hesitation and guaranteeing haphazard instruction. For most men, bluffing their way along the road to competence seemed almost second nature. However, for many women used to reading instructions, asking questions, and proceeding cautiously, it was mind-boggling. Anatomy was a good testing ground because mistakes there didn't matter, but the mental resolve required to saw through a skull was the same as that I called upon later on to plunge a needle into a living patient.

On balance, I think that learning to stretch your abilities to the utmost is one of the most valuable benefits of a medical education. I am no longer as afraid of failure as I was as an undergraduate. I believe that I will always be as good as the next guy at the same level of skill, and diligence and hard work are far more important than talent. This self-confidence is almost palpable. I am reminded of the night a group of my close women friends from medical school met at a small restaurant. We were at the end of our residencies, seven years removed from the timid freshmen who clung to one another for support. As we stood waiting for our table, six forthright and obviously self-assured young women, a patron at the bar, moderately inebriated, leaned over and asked, "Are you astronauts?"

There is no free lunch, however. The price of soul-stretching is constant feelings of inadequacy and moments of sheer terror. The first year is a wrenching transition from student (read dilettante) to apprentice. Anatomy draws you out of the books into the lab. The course work is onerous, crowding the conscious hours and spilling into the unconscious. Your vocabulary expands by several thousand words, the equivalent of a new language. And time plays tricks, expanding in the middle of the quarter so that courses seem endless, but snapping back to flit by as the quarters pass. I used to joke that by the end of the first week I had invested so much in medical school that I could never quit; I was being only partly facetious. The husband of a friend from medical school claimed that the only time in his law training that he felt truly obsessed was when he was studying for the bar, but complained that his wife routinely hallucinated histology slides in the clouds as soon as she started her training.

When I looked back at college from the perspective of medical school, it seemed as though I must have wasted a tremendous amount of time. I rarely took more than two science courses at a time, and since geology labs were usually field trips, my life-style was closer to that of a humanities concentrator than of a biologist. Nine o'clock classes were beyond the call of duty; I even knew people who flunked early courses because they couldn't wake up. Well, my first-year medical school schedule had an eight o'clock class four days a week. Trudging up the hill to that class became a symbol of true grit in our household. It was the year of the energy crisis, when the government tried instituting daylight savings time in the winter. We watched the sun rise from histology lab. Every course had labs; anatomy's were two entire afternoons a week. I probably spent more time in class in the first quarter than I did my entire first year of college.

My undergraduate years were divided into semesters, with generous reading periods to catch up before exams. It was a system geared to the gentleman scholar. My medical school rushed along on a quarter schedule. Since each course had two or three midterms and a final, testing started several weeks rather than several months into the term. There was no such thing as missing a few days or catching up later. My dissecting group argued over whether we needed to spend both Saturday and Sunday afternoons in the lab, finally agreeing to do some work individually since I, for one, was adamantly opposed to ruining the entire weekend.

The odd thing was, the professors seemed always available also. Saturday review sessions were commonplace, and labs never formally ended. Coming from a college where the average undergraduate had little personal contact with faculty, I was astounded by the access we had to professors. It would have been easy to spend every waking hour studying; I didn't, but I was not at the top of my class, either. During the week I could psych myself into preparing for the next day, staying up until midnight every night if necessary, but Fridays I fell apart. I would sleep from seven P.M. Friday to noon Saturday, from a combination of exhaustion and depression. I hasten to add that my experience was not universal. I was running scared at first, still worried that I would be unmasked as a humanist impostor by the next test. My husband, who had a much stronger science background, managed to adhere more closely to his undergraduate pattern of cramming before tests. Given the number of tests, however, even his freedom was sharply curtailed.

By and large, I thought our professors were reasonably tolerant of the women and minority students in the class. It was as though once the walls of the club had been breached, they decided to accept the intruders in good faith. We had our share of lecturers who discussed "pregnancy in man" and more than our share of classroom confrontations over semantic sexism. Once when a female student wrote the address of the women's group meeting on the blackboard, a male student scrawled an announcement, The Men's Group

Will Be Meeting at the Bar, just below. In general, I would estimate there was as much hostility from our peers as from the professors. Some white men insisted that minority students were taking places away from other white men. In fact, due to the expansion of medical schools in the 1960s and 1970s, the nationwide increase in minority enrollment was accomplished without decreasing the numbers of white students, but such facts fell on deaf ears.

Tolerance evaporated when it came to those who fell behind academically. A friend who took summer anatomy reported that, after the first test, the professor congratulated the class as a whole then read a list of students who were to stay after class to discuss their grades. He remembers how shocked he was; failure in undergraduate work had always been a private matter. Failing a course in medical school often means losing the whole year, since courses are rarely offered twice, and at least at my school there was a strict prerequisite system. Histology, the microscopic anatomy of normal tissue, was a prerequisite for pathology, the microscopic anatomy of abnormal tissue. Physiology was a prerequisite to the introduction of clinical medicine. The National Board Exam Part I was a prerequisite for starting on the wards third year.

There were two ways to perceive this rigid lock-step system. I preferred to believe that my professors had high standards because they really wanted to turn out good doctors and I enjoyed the personal attention. Others characterized the system more succinctly as jail. It certainly had that aspect. I vividly recall the shock of the fresh air as I descended that hill after anatomy lab, darkness already falling. Most nights, I made a ritual stop at an organic-food store. The smell of formalin that had permeated my clothes through the lab coat clashed with the fruity incense of the shelves. Dazed, I would wander through, marveling at the texture of the grains, the colors of the vegetables, and the aroma of the fruits. I might buy an apple to excuse my presence, but I went there not to purchase but to recharge my sensory batteries. It was my reentry chamber from the land of the dead to the land of the living.

One day some of us sat at lunch in the cafeteria and compared notes on our experience. Nightmares were routine, we discovered. Some nightmares were quite involved, like a Boston woman's dream of meeting an anatomy professor as a minister in Old South Church and watching him stir a bowl of jewels until two eyeballs emerged. Others were fiercely direct: a friend dreamed that she was a gazelle bounding across the plains with her herd until she was gunned down by hunters in white coats. Another student studying for his final in head and neck anatomy, where dissection is performed on heads separated from their bodies, dreamed that students themselves were beheaded as they entered the exam. The other students didn't seem to mind losing their bodies; all the heads were lined up cheerfully spouting the answers to the questions of the exam.

I learned too late to do me any good that there is a considerable body of sociological research dealing with initiation rites, and with medical students in particular. There are also counseling resources, academic and emotional, at every medical school. I recommend pursuing such help early on if the first year seems overwhelming; the pace only accelerates. However, I would warn against confiding personal difficulties to academic figures, even those with benign titles such as Dean of Students. Four years later, when professors are called upon to write your recommendation for internship, they will think of those early conversations, even if they make no mention of them in writing.

After all, the loyalty of a dean is to an institution, not to an individual. Your medical school hopes to make a reasonable return on its investment in you: You should graduate, whether or not graduating is in your best interest. So for academic problems, seek out the dean. For the cosmic question What am I doing here? you deserve the privileged confidentiality of the therapist-patient relationship. And just think! All psychiatrists went to medical school and, chances are, they weren't crazy about it.

Other than anatomy, the courses of the first year resemble undergraduate science courses. The difference is that the quantity of material presented mounts and mounts, like overleavened bread dough. Out of this morass of facts rises the one gigantic question that sprawls over the clinical years. It rears its head during the introductory lectures and pops up every other day thereafter. How much of this stuff do we have to know to practice? Is our performance in these classes critical to the development of medical skills? Do these grades count for internship? And if we do have to learn all this material, how?

Everyone had a different opinion. Those who had been humanities concentrators as undergraduates clung to claims of some classmates that none of the basic science courses matters. Those who had taken biochemistry before and were breezing through the second time around maintained that the course was crucial to later clinical understanding. Although most of us were grateful for the pass-fail-honors system instituted the year before our class entered, there was one out-front career pre-med who rocked our first class meeting by announcing that he not only wanted to keep the honors designation, instead of moving to a totally pass-fail system, but he wished we could return to grades. He had set his sights on an internship at Massachusetts General

Hospital and intended to step over as many bodies as necessary to get there. (He made it.)

I can't tell you what you'll need to know as a practicing physician. Much depends on the field you choose. As an internist I can get by with an approximate knowledge of anatomy most of the time. As a radiologist or a surgeon, I couldn't. Pharmacology, by contrast, is crucial to me and fairly irrelevant to a radiologist. As a rule of thumb, the more general your practice, the more information it would be useful to retain from the first two years. Note the phrase "it would be useful." You can't remember everything you're taught. The saving grace is that the important principles and facts will be repeated over and over again during your training. Even the lectures addressed to fellows in their fourth year of post-medical school training typically start with a review of the anatomy or physiology of the organ in question. So do the continuing education lectures I attend.

Along the way to private practice, however, you will encounter many a clinical professor who will expect you to have this or that fact at the tip of your tongue. You also have to pass board exams on this material. So it is not enough simply to lie back and absorb just enough to pass the tests, counting on hearing it again. You have to keep pushing, to retain just a little more, especially if facts slip past you quickly. But remember, medicine is a vast jigsaw puzzle without edges. You won't ever finish learning, but the more pieces you fit in any particular area, the simpler placing the next pieces will become.

Nothing will protect you from professors out to "pump" you for trivia. As a third-year resident I presented a case in front of several rheumatologists, in which I had to refer to a joint in the toe that I hadn't thought about since

29

anatomy seven years before. I named it by analogy to the comparable joint in the hand, which was a good guess, but wrong. Since I was pointing to the joint on the patient's foot and the analogy was correct, the five or six doctors in the room knew what I meant. Yet one of them stared at me with the fake bewilderment familiar to anyone who has ever used the wrong definite article in front of a perfectly pronounced noun while speaking French. You know they understand, but it's more important to them to make you feel like a fool than to communicate. The rest of the doctors corrected me and proceeded to discuss the case.

As a senior resident I could view that one doctor's reaction to my faux pas as his problem. The student, under constant evaluation, cannot afford such complacency. All your work counts toward internship. It is true that the preclinical work counts less, unless you're heading for a research career, but since it's the underpinning of the clinical work, you can't expect to loaf for two years and make up for it by shining the next two. There is no point in castigating yourself if you don't do as well initially as you expected, however. All the people taking chemistry for cultural enrichment are off in law school now, leaving you with the hardcore fanatics. It's no accident that the performance on the MCAT correlates with academic success in the preclinical years. Those students aren't necessarily brighter; they've just seen the material before.

If you start to fall seriously behind, don't make the mistake of skipping lectures or labs to study at home. Lectures may be an inefficient way to assimilate material, especially if, like me, you can't learn a phone number without seeing it written. The problem is that medical school affords little of the anonymity you may have cherished in undergraduate days. Your absence is noted, particularly if you are one of a few women or minority students. Attendance is considered central to a good-faith effort to catch up. So be there.

The student who is not in academic difficulty often decides that it is not worth his while to show up for every lecture. At some schools there are organized note collectives, so only a few students need attend any given class. They take the notes and copy them for the rest of the students. Most of our professors, bowing to student pressure, prepared comprehensive handouts that also rendered attendance optional. I tended to go to class partly because, in the words of my husband, I am a "goody-goody girl." He missed many lectures, especially second year, and did just as well. Some of my motivation for going to school was social. I couldn't square off with the books all day as well as all night. Toward the end of my second year, I was also feeling sorry for the lecturers. They were presenting their life's work to 30 students out of a class of 150. A few would bitterly berate those of us who did show up for the absence of our fellows. The next time they addressed fewer still. The problem of how to present the necessary material in an interesting manner is a fundamental one.

One stratagem the student can adopt to counteract the tedium of lecture-lab-lecture-lecture is to enroll in any clinical elective offered: courses such as surface anatomy, where the bones and muscles are demonstrated on volunteers from the audience, or beginning radiology, or best of all, a preceptorship with a physician in the community, reinforce the material in a dramatic fashion. Not to speak of the advantage of standing up once in a while. All that attentive sitting is hard on the hams.

Many schools also have some sort of required clinical exposure during the first year. We were assigned to a senior resident one afternoon a week, and stumbled through hospital corridors for a few hours. The content of these clinical glimpses was negligible, since we had no concept of disease processes. But my resident, a woman, quickly became a role model, and I lost some of my fears of smelly, sick people. Medical educators who evaluate such things call time so spent useless. But I think they tend to forget just how raw their recruits are. I remember the lunch hour scramble to our basement lockers to ditch books and grab white coats and stethoscopes. Once a shy classmate a few lockers down, clearly as nervous as I, asked me to straighten his tie. As I was doing so, he realized what an intimacy the anxiety of the moment had prompted and he blushed deeply. He had asked a stranger to groom him as a mother or lover would, because the need to make a good impression was greater than social convention. The beginning of camaraderie.

As the first year ends, the unwary students who have not lifted their noses from the cadavers the whole time find themselves confronted with what may well be the last summer vacation they will ever know. By all means, take advantage of it. Don't start work the week after exams. And quit before you have to return to school. You deserve a vacation; you just finished your first year.

3

THE
REAL WORLD

At one point during orientation week at my medical school, a psychologist distributed questionnaires that were to be used in a study of how the attitudes of medical students evolve over the four years of their studies. We were asked to predict how our own views would change. She instructed us to answer the questions without regard to our hopes or fears, just to try to imagine our thoughts four years hence. After the papers were collected, she volunteered that most freshman students worried that they would become conservative, insensitive, and avaricious, but that previous studies had shown only that students become more decisive. I have never checked her sources, nor do I know what became of her questionnaires, one of so many we dutifully completed in the maze of social science. I suspected at the time that her words reflected more empathy than fact, but I assumed that four years later I would at least be able to identify how medical school had changed me.

In making that assumption, I forgot that medical students, like all human beings, live and grow within a social milieu of which medical school is only a part, albeit a hefty chunk. Over the ensuing years, I became a different person. I made new friends, I married, I learned to backpack, I took Spanish lessons, I started jogging. I explored most of the West Coast, I read *The Golden Notebook,* I tried therapy. Above all, I aged: A twenty-five-year-old requires a different refraction, even for rose-colored glasses, than a twenty-one-year-old. I have referred earlier to the problems that arise at the interface of medical school and real life. In this chapter I want to start to address some of these problems, since the integration of boot camp into the home is probably the greatest challenge the aspiring doctor faces. And whatever emerges from the chrysalis at the end of four years has as much to do with the ability of the organism to adapt as it does with school indoctrination.

Why does medical school present such a problem? Why is the suicide rate so high among medical students and, later, among doctors? Or in broader sociological terms, why do these students in particular have notoriously more difficulty maintaining relationships with significant others? There has been ample speculation on these points but I would like to add my own two cents worth.

First, I can think of few professions that require such intensive work for so long for such remote rewards. This contention is only valid in its entirety. For instance, it may well take a young lawyer five years after law school, years of overtime and a driven life-style, to become established. Perhaps even longer. But from his or her second year of law school on, he or she can obtain jobs that approximate the work of a full-fledged lawyer—and be paid for this work. And law school does not require thirty-six-hour shifts in a hospital.

The medical student without a doctor in the family can only guess at the life of a practicing physician for at least five years of his or her training. Part-time work is next to impossible because of time constraints, and if such work is available it cannot be in the role of a physician outside the teaching institution. In the past few years, courses in ambulatory medicine, created to capture federal grants, have attempted to introduce the student to the real world of outpatient care, but I wonder if they have been any more successful nationwide than they were at my institution. The patients included the dregs of humanity, malingerers, schizophrenics, drug abusers, since anyone else would not have escaped the jealous tentacles of the private sector. And we were required to accost them in interdisciplinary teams (the terms of the grant, of course) consisting of a medical student, a pharmacy student, a nursing student, and sometimes even a dental student. That course made even the most stalwart clinicians-to-be have second thoughts. There is also an interesting financial consideration that promises to remove medical students even further from patient responsibility. Insurance carriers and government agencies are beginning to withhold payment for services that are not performed by a licensed physician. While I am certain that the intent of such a policy is to correct abuses of the system, the effort may well be to relegate the junior physician to the role of a glorified medical assistant.

The medical student works harder for four years than the law student for three but will not earn a competitive salary until finished with house-staff training. During the last year of my residency, the seventh year of my postcollege training, I earned less than my lawyer sister did on her first job her fourth year out of college. Not to speak of the starting salaries of M.B.A.s. Certainly physicians can make more money eventually. But I submit that it is precisely because that potential earning power is the only comprehensible reward to the student enmeshed in an apparently endless hierarchy of onerous training that money often becomes the primary motivation of the previously idealistic student. Making more money begins to seem like the only way to make up for those lost years of adulthood, for deferral of childbearing, for the years of watching college classmates move ahead financially and psychologically. It is not just the students who learn to think of money first. Spouses who resent never being able to plan an outing and long-suffering parents who seek reflected glory or grandchildren begin to look toward the time when "at least they'll be making money."

In all fairness, I must acknowledge that many entering medical students seek a prolongation of adolescence. College wasn't so bad, after all, and the idea of more of a known quantity in a structured environment seems comfortable compared to the business of selling oneself for a job. To a senior in college, the freedom of the working world can be obscured by the anxiety of choice. To the dissatisfied graduate working at an unfulfilling job a few years out, the prospect of further education opens as a refuge for the battered soul.

Well, medical school isn't college. And sooner or later, in a quiet moment of honesty, most medical students realize that they are as ready as they are going to be for adulthood. They are tired of the faculty controlling their lives, fixing the horizontal and the vertical. They realize that the cold, real world looks refreshing from the medical school hot-house. And worse, one day the student meets a resident or fellow who is looking for a job and realizes that the M.D. degree is no more a ticket to personal satisfaction than the B.A. was. This quiet moment usually comes too late for the rational student to abandon medical studies.

The less introspective student may be driven to the quiet moment by an impatient spouse who, after all, didn't sign on the dotted line but suffers the indignities of unpredictable long hours and capricious instructors as they are reflected in the couple's newly restricted life-style. A college reunion where everyone else's job seems glamorous and well paid may jolt the student's self-image. Students who are alone wonder if they will ever have the time to establish a relationship with another person; women over thirty worry that they will have to choose between their training and children. Once the white jacket begins to chafe, there seems no end to vulnerable flesh.

Here begins the advice. Allow yourself an outlet for doubt. Seek this outlet during the first two years when constant drudgery discourages you: Once the clinical work begins, questions of competence can quickly produce an internal crisis. You may be fortunate enough to live with someone who will allow you to talk about your life as a medical student, but in my experience this is very rare. It is difficult enough for a significant other to put up with the hours of loneliness without having then to listen to your complaints when you finally arrive home. The universal answer is, "Well, why the hell did you get yourself into this?" followed by, "Don't talk about medicine on *our* time, there is little enough of it as it is." Even if you live with another student, as I did, that person is not going to be able to wrestle with your angst for fear of slipping into the morass himself.

Your parents are of little help. If they are doctors themselves, they may respond with the convenient amnesia of those who have already passed through the initiation rites. Besides, only a truly ungrateful wretch would share all his thoughts about quitting school with those financing the endeavor. Money is at the root of most marital discussions about school as well, since the non-medical student spouse is often supporting the student. I have seen a pattern develop among certain couples in which the newly assertive wife literally stops any conversation verging on medicine with "I'm slaving to put you there, so shut up." Such an attitude is hardly liberated, just cruel and shortsighted— shortsighted because at school that man will certainly find women willing to listen. And cruel because it represents the new physician's great double bind: You are expected to act in a superhuman fashion, to work endlessly, never to complain, and to be eternally cheerful in exhaustion, yet remain humble and even apologetic about your work.

When I was a medical student, I studied once a week with a small group of women. While we did cover coursework, our most valuable service to each other was as a sounding board for doubts and fears we could not express easily elsewhere, even to our supportive significant others. I think for many students such study groups, even on a more informal basis, can be a valuable outlet. I had never studied in groups before because I was always too compulsive myself to suffer those who hadn't prepared. One joy of medical school was the discovery that almost everyone in my class was as compulsive as I, if not more so, so such group sessions could be quite productive. Even with other students, though, I think the key to successful relationships is not to expect any one person to absorb the burbling effluent of your medical school experiences. In other intense learning and socialization situations—and I return to the military for the analogy of boot camp—the students are separated from home, so no outsider has to endure the day-by-day crises of stress. Paradoxically, such separation may be healthier for relationships than sharing the experience. It is no fun to watch your lover study for a midterm every week, to receive only absentminded attention yourself.

Which brings up the whole question of how to arrange your life so that the person who shares it is as little agitated as possible. Planning for the other person should begin before you apply to medical school so that mutually compatible cities with reasonable jobs or school opportunities for the other person can be identified. Once the acceptance has dictated the city, you should try to live in an area where the nonstudent has easy access to amusements and friends. A cheap apartment on the outskirts of town is not worth it if there will be only one car and transportation is poor. The non-medical student will have an enormous amount of time alone on nights and weekends when you are studying, not to speak of entire days you will be absent during the clinical years. If that time is filled waiting for you, the relationship will not survive, period. Perhaps in years past there were women willing to wait years, but no longer. And no man would consider it.

In order to shore up a relationship for the stresses to come, I would suggest that the medical student resolve to put aside inviolate couple time as soon as the schedule for the semester is established. This luxury of certainty is only possible for the first two years, so take advantage of it. Plan to get away the one weekend that isn't followed by a midterm and identify the days that can be preserved whole. Analyze your weekdays to determine the time of day you are most amenable to company. Are you the kind of person who can drop the biochemistry book and make love at eleven P.M.? My husband is, but I'm not, so we found that the late afternoon hours, which we tended to waste anyway since neither of us could launch right into studying after class, were the best time for us to talk and conduct the business of life. After dinner, we could study without worrying that the other one had been ignored all day.

The non-medical students, for their part, must work at developing interests that they can pursue alone. Those who have demanding jobs themselves (many men but, unfortunately, not so many women) are a step ahead of the game. They can work late with impunity most of the time, as long as they try to coordinate their free days with yours. Even if such coordination is not always possible, which is frequently the case, two busy people seem to be happier than couples in which one is busy and the other isn't. If there are children, the burden of childcare usually falls entirely on the person not in medical school and can be barely tolerable. Every couple has to work that problem out for themselves, depending on the ages of the children and the distribution of responsibilities that existed before medical school, but I think this is the one instance where the partner in medical school is just going to have to work even harder. I had a friend who used to wake up at five A.M. on weekends to finish studying before his wife awoke— gallant beyond the call of duty, I thought. But with children, your time is not your own, and the bizarre home stratagems, with inevitably less sleep, may be the only solution.

Many campuses have so-called Exchanges: formerly, and still largely, wives' auxiliaries, which can be very helpful for the woman with children in providing baby-sitters and activities to get her out of the house. The drawback of these organizations is that the other members are also involved with medicine, so that the competitive gossip and speculation that permeate the medical student's world can become the whole family's social milieu. For some young couples, this is logical, even desirable, but other couples, particularly those in which the man is not in medicine, quickly find that the question of whether to socialize with other students is a true test of the relationship.

My husband and I were medical students in the same class and we moved across the country to attend the school of our choice. Obviously, we made friends within the class: Whom else did we know or have time to get to know? Other couples who do not move may already have a social circle that will continue to accept the medical student in his or her new role. Most couples end up seeing some students socially, generally to the discomfort of the non-medical student who complains that all the students do is talk about school. No question but that this is true, and for two reasons. School takes up most of the students' working hours and they usually don't know each other, at least initially, on any other level. It's not any different from a group of other professionals who work intensely together, but medical training just lasts so much longer. Some women are content to have their own conversation in such gatherings, but men generally react by limiting their medical student partners to a few such affairs, refusing to attend the others.

A medical student myself, I was still uncomfortable at such parties, because, as a woman, I didn't belong to the old-boy network or see the world in the same way as many of my fellow students. Their wives were busy having babies, an option I felt was not open to me during training. I often felt I belonged to a third gender, neither male nor pregnant. The male-student friends we made did not have career-minded wives, which may have been an accident, but I suspect not. The traditional arrangement of one overa-chiever per family eases the tricky business of establishing intracouple priorities, and M.D.s still are financially secure enough that two salaries are not mandatory.

Friends outside medicine used to comment, "It must be easier for you both to be in medicine." Yes and no. It was easier because we did not constantly have to explain or defend our hours, our exhaustion. It was harder because often neither one of us had the time or energy to plan outings or to shop for dinner. We were more strapped financially than the couples with a salary and, fundamen-tally, there was just no respite from school. On the other hand, I felt lucky compared to my single women friends who had no warm body and no energy to look for one. Not to speak of the stigmas of brains and potential earnings attached to the woman doctor, which make socializing so difficult. The few intraclass romances I was privy to ended disastrously, partly because the academic competition, which was a strain for an established relationship like mine, proved too divisive for new couples.

As I have suggested earlier, women living with men out-side of medicine fared little better than single women. Dur-ing the increasing feminist awareness of the past few years, sex-role reversals have often displayed most sharply the privileges men have assumed, and women granted, uncon-sciously. Just the thought of a male nurse, a house husband, or female car mechanic challenges us to redefine those roles outside a sexual context. Only as I watched my women friends fend off the demands of their husbands did I realize how little wives have asserted themselves in such situations.

One man, who was unemployed, refused to move ten miles into the city to spare his medical student partner the commute and ultimately made it so impossible for her to study by constantly demanding attention that she came to live in her own apartment in the city, staying with him only on vacations. That relationship has endured, by the way, and she finished medical school, no thanks to him. Another woman never took an elective course so that she could spend her time taking care of her stepdaughter on our elective day. Would a man have felt similarly compelled? I doubt it. Another woman would announce in the middle of our scheduled study group, "Well, I have to go now. Danny wants me home earlier." Or he would call, summoning her home. Most telling of all, conversations with these men were dominated by pseudosympathetic exclamations, such as, "I don't know why she puts up with it. I keep telling her it's not worth it." I never heard a woman express those feelings. However difficult life appeared at any given time, however much the women complained, on a fundamental level they gave their men the benefit of the doubt. It's the same old story: "Sure, you can discover the cure for cancer, honey. Just leave me clean underwear."

To be complete, I should mention the life of the single male medical student. He may well be the most sought-after male in society. I used to love to walk around the hospital with an available male intern. From the cafeteria to the morgue, his way was smoothed by female smiles and gracious alacrity that evaporated when I was alone. Now I happen to know several guys who weren't happy with the playboy life they were offered, who longed to settle down, but it must have been an ego boost anyway. My friend Rachel, a single medical student with the ultimate Jewish mother, reports a conversation they had her first year. Her mother was bubbling over with news of a hot prospect: good family, good-looking, and, best of all, he was "going to be a doctor!" Rachel countered, "But, Mom, *I'm* going to be a doctor." It just wasn't the same.

Before I leave the outside world, I want to mention a problem I never thought would arise during the first two years but popped up right after registration. That is the family assumption that you are now qualified to give medical advice in every area. This is a generous assumption for a licensed physician, but it is ludicrous for a first-year medical student. You can't even read the journal articles if you wanted to look up the problem. The best strategy to handle these medical questions, even when they occur late in your training, is to help the family members find trustworthy physicians with impeccable credentials and trust them. It is impossible to second-guess a physician based on a patient's understanding of the problem, especially when the patient is a parent. And you are in no position to manage a case yourself from a thousand miles away. Although this advice seems perfectly obvious as I write it, I learned it as a house officer when I heard a full professor talking about his mother, who was ill. As he pointed out, we would call it malpractice if a strange doctor was giving long-distance advice about a patient he'd only met socially. Your role should be to serve as an intelligent ear, and in serious cases, you can help both the doctor and the family by calling at crisis points and helping to explain the necessity of an operation and the futility of further treatment. But even that comes later. As a first-year student, answer honestly, "I really don't know anything about primary biliary cirrhosis, and you are better off trusting your doctor or obtaining a formal second opinion from another physician." They won't believe you, you'll feel cruel and helpless, but it's the truth.

4

SECOND YEAR: STUDENT MEETS PATIENT

A few months into the second year, a first-year student whom you know from undergraduate days or meet in the cafeteria will ask you, "Is it better in the second year?" Hassled by a new set of courses and new clinical responsibilities, you will be tempted to answer no, for you feel you're working just as hard as last year. But if you look at your friend's face long enough to remember how overwhelming it all seemed last year, you'll answer more honestly, "Well, it's different. Not necessarily easier, but different."

At most schools, the second-year curriculum changes toward the clinical: histology becomes physiology, biochemistry and anatomy give way to pharmacology and microbiology. For some students this is a relief, for others, who would rather memorize a static system than try to integrate the change of a dynamic one, the new courses can be an unwelcome challenge. Then, too, after a summer's vacation, just the resumption of the routine of study is irksome. You feel you know the other members of your class all too well, those who will ask the stupid question just on the hour and cut into the ten-minute break; the sycophantic crew in the front row always asking for more references, as though you had time to read anything extra. The adrenaline that launched you into the first year isn't there in the same amount. After all, you passed everything last year, there's no reason to believe you won't again.

The year under your belt is a strength as well as a liability, of course. You thought you knew how to study when you entered medical school, but your mind is like a laser beam now compared to the twenty-five watt incandescent bulb you started with last year. You have learned to approach a page of gobbledygook and to extract the kernel of information you need. This skill will serve you well in all your medical training but may temporarily impair your ability to read fiction or poetry. I found when turning to fiction I consciously had to downshift my concentration to prevent myself from bulldozing through, looking for the facts to memorize. On the other hand, long nonfiction articles Scientific American or The New Yorker became more accessible. Next to medical writing, any other style seems a model of lucidity.

I think you'll also find that even after a summer off your endurance is better. The long days are almost second nature, and you can judge with precision how much you need to stoke the afterburners to propel you through any particular minute. The studying, then, as long as you have the patience for it, should not be a problem: It's an old game by now.

The new year is the clinical work. At my school, the

course was called Introduction to Clinical Medicine, but whatever the name, it is the first clinical course that counts, the one where physical diagnosis is taught: how to interview a patient or "take a history," in medical jargon, how to examine each organ system, and how to interpret your findings in order to figure out what is wrong with the patient or at least narrow down the possibilities to formulate a "differential diagnosis."

This is bread-and-butter medicine, the foundation of your clinical work from this time forward. If you don't learn to examine a patient, think through the case, and present it cogently to someone else, you'll not only find yourself having trouble the rest of your clinical training, but you'll be a mediocre doctor. A layman reading this might think you wouldn't be much of a doctor at all, but he would be underestimating the role of rote in medical training. Most doctors muddle through by learning what tests to order for any given complaint and following up the abnormals. They also refer quickly when a problem does not fall within their specialty. If they don't trust their own exams, they just call in a consultant. A urologist doesn't listen to the heart, except to record its presence. And I've watched internists order stomach X rays for a young woman with nausea and vomiting rather than run a pregnancy test.

The reason I'm mentioning all this is that I didn't know any of it my second year. I thought I had to learn every aspect of physical diagnosis right then and there, and that if I didn't I would be killing people right and left. And, at least among my friends, this seemed to be a fairly common delusion, which was reinforced by our instructors. The surgeon who teaches the rectal exam emphasizes the danger of missing the diagnosis of cancer, the cardiologist describes what would happen to a patient with undiagnosed valvular heart disease, the opthalmologist dwells on the importance of seeing microaneurysms in order to make the diagnosis of diabetes. They are all correct, but unless you plan to practice in the hinterlands or a Third World country, you will not be called upon to be an expert in every subspecialty. And if you do choose to practice in the bush, being able to make such sophisticated diagnoses won't help your patients who are dying of malnutrition and infection before they are old enough to develop other problems.

I don't mean to suggest that you shouldn't try to hit every ball you're pitched. Everything you learn now will save you time and trouble later on. Just remember that you can't learn it all—certainly not the first time you hear it— and that most of your instructors are specialists. Nor should you feel intimidated by your classmates. You will find, to your amazement, that while you are struggling to distinguish a systolic murmur from a diastolic murmur, some of your peers will claim to hear three kinds of murmurs in a single patient, after the instructor has described them. By and large, these students are bluffing. I was silent quite often. I knew I couldn't hear the second murmur, much less the third, straining as hard as I could. But when I was one of four students listening to a patient who had often not even been asked if he would mind our exams until we were crowded in the room, and the other three students were nodding sagely, I could only hold out for so long. I might ask once if the instructor could describe or locate the murmur again, but I wouldn't ask twice, whether I heard it or not. That was my own code of honor, to ask once. Some students would persist longer, others never asked. By my code, those who held up the lesson lost sight of the patient, while those who pretended to catch on to everything right away were dishonest. Yet who can say what the proper etiquette of group examination is?

Consider the patient. One of my greatest weaknesses as a medical student and greatest strengths as a doctor is my ability to perceive the patient as a human being. It is not that difficult, after all, to tell if a modest women is embarrassed to have a group feel the lump in her breast or if a patient tires taking deep breaths or if the fourth abdominal exam hurts while the first was merely uncomfortable. I did not try to empathize. I tried not to, since my job was to learn to examine, not to think. Most of the time my colleagues seemed to have no difficulty concentrating on the task at hand, but I was always offering a gown or taking less time than I needed to hear the pneumonia rattle. All silently, of course, for I was no heroine. I could not interrupt a lecture or small group session to say that the patient needed a rest. I would compare notes later with my study group friends and find that we often shared the same feeling of impotence and anxiety in our clinical sessions, but none of us spoke out. We needed the skill being demonstrated, and we needed the approval and the grade of the instructor.

Much later, it has occurred to me that my problem might have been more a failure to identify with the instructor than any particular empathy with the patient who, after all, I didn't know and generally would never see again. I could not throw myself heart and soul into the doctor role, for I was too conscious of being merely the student using, if not exploiting, the patients for my own experience. It did not salve my conscience to note that a disproportionate number of clinic patients were poor and members of ethnic minorities. While this consciousness was an annoyance at group sessions, it provoked stronger conflicts when we were sent to interview patients on our own.

Many years later, I still consider those first solo patient examinations the moral equivalent of being thrown to the lions. Let me set the scene at my medical school: After a nine-hour day of classes, you would check the bulletin board to learn your patient assignment. Once the assignments were posted, you usually had two days to find the patient, take the history, perform the physical, and write it up, although these were class days like any other, of course. So the first struggle was logistically whether to go home and eat dinner then return more rested, or plunge on until you were finished and have dinner late. Whichever you chose, people at home wouldn't see much of you those evenings, since a typical student exam would take several hours. Seizing the time, you would locate the ward in question and ask the ward secretary where Mr. Smith might be found. It was safest to identify yourself right away, particularly if you were a woman, so you'd start out, "Hello, my name is Jane Albers and I'm a second-year medical student looking for Clarence Smith." The ward secretary would look you up and down with undisguised scorn and point to Room 612, often admonishing, "He's had a lot of tests today, he may not be up to a physical." Grinning wanly, you would shuffle down the hall burdened with opthalmoscope, stethoscope, and enough neurological paraphernalia to supply a small clinic, not to speak of a pocket manual of physical diagnosis in case the patient articulated a complaint for which you could not remember the exam.

The door would be open, depriving you of the chance to knock and announce yourself properly, so you would knock and walk in at the same time. There you would find either that the patient was on the bedpan, in which case he would ask you to take it if you were a woman (read, automatically, nurse), or that the entire Georgia branch of the family whom he had not seen in twenty years had crowded into the room and would be looking at you suspiciously. Both situations challenged your doctor role.

My advice in the first situation is, don't take the bedpan, no matter how strong your feelings against the ward hierarchy. You will not change the fact that nurses and orderlies are oppressed by taking the bedpan, nor will you spare them work since as soon as you take it you will realize that you have no idea what to do with it. Besides, what you *will* do is convince the patient that you *are* a nurse and your interview will suffer.

The question of the family's right to visit versus your right to time with the patient is a deeper philosophical one. You are within your rights to ask the family to leave the room. At this point, the patient will protest, "But three people examined me yesterday. And I'm leaving tomorrow." And he's right. He was examined by a resident, an intern, and a medical student on the ward team. If you have committed yourself to asking them to leave, you must proceed solely on the authority of your presence, because you have no logical argument to counter his. Your exam will be long, inexpert, and thoroughly irrelevant to his care. Another option is to capitulate entirely and leave until visiting hours are over. This is generally a tremendous inconvenience to you and your family. You can come back tomorrow, but the relatives may also be back and your deadline will be that much closer.

So far I have only described the recalcitrant patient. There are also patients who will refuse outright, moaning that they are sick and can't be bothered. One patient told a friend he didn't want "no nigger doctor." Other patients have gone professional after multiple hospitalizations, so they spout diagnoses instead of symptoms. Perhaps the worst patient for the hapless student is the nonstop talker with head-to-toe complaints. I used to agonize about politely cutting off patients until I realized that subtlety is lost on a true hypochondriac. Acknowledge his concerns with a phrase—"I understand you've had quite a bit of trouble with your hemorrhoids over the years"—then change the subject—"But I don't believe you mentioned when your chest pain started." And keep doing it.

One student in my class bawled out patients as though they were petulant children, emphasizing that they had no choice since they had signed into a teaching hospital. Such arrogance won that student a prestigious internship but not the respect of his peers. On the other hand, the student who retreats entirely will never learn to be a clinician, which, after all, involves learning to approach all sorts of human beings. You must believe in yourself as a doctor to get the job done. I do not advise advertising yourself as "Doctor" Albers before graduation, however. Patients are not stupid, and they will see right through you. Many states now have laws requiring that your medical student status be clear on your name tag to avoid just such deception.

When will you feel like a doctor? Probably about half-way through your internship, when you have developed enough judgment to begin to function autonomously. To a second-year student, that time can seem remote. Again, give yourself a break. You don't become an M.D. overnight emotionally, any more than you do intellectually. Perhaps you are learning that you are not cut out to be a clinician, and that's good to learn early rather than late.

Even for those who eventually opt for clinical medicine, it takes time to grow into the role. I think most of my classmates shared my unthinking assumption that patients would be people pretty much like ourselves, with the same expectations of the medical system and a concern for their own welfare. We recognized that there would be ethnic diversity and even language barriers, but we thought that, deep down, people would react similarly when ill. Nothing could be further from the truth. Oh, there are cultural patterns that emerge pretty quickly and are predictable enough to inspire racist jokes. But there's no accounting for what the psychiatrists list as "insight and judgment" on the mental status exam. I've seen hypereducated patients who had none and laborers who grasped the essence of their medical problem immediately, if not the fancy terms. Forty-year-old executives faint receiving the same shot that a ten-year-old manages with aplomb. Belligerence, non-compliance, and self-destructive behavior know no socio-economic barriers.

When I started medical school, I thought I wanted to be an obstetrician and gynecologist. I knew it was a field that "needed" more women, and I had visions of myself treating and educating women like myself and my friends who sought to make informed decisions about birth control and plan the joyous deliveries of our healthy children. I quickly learned how very privileged I was to even consider such issues. Far from seeing the pill as a plot against women, as some feminists contend, my patients saw it as synony-mous with birth control: They would as soon insert a dia-phragm in their vaginas as fly to the moon. On my obstetrics rotation I watched high-risk deliveries of premature infants from teen-age mothers who had no self-concept, much less thoughts about motherhood or parenting. Well, that was a clinic population, not representative of medicine in the suburbs. True enough. But did I go to medical school to retreat to the suburbs? I did spend one day with an obste-trician in private practice. He had an excellent reputation, but he whipped through his patients like a whirlwind, greeting each woman in the stirrups and leaving no time for discussion. He was obliging, though: He agreed to ma-nipulate the contraceptive prescription for a woman who wanted to attend an est seminar where she would not be allowed to go to the bathroom and wanted her period delayed for a week.

As I rotated services in the last two years, I learned as much about people as about medicine. I found that, by and large, the foibles of humanity amused and fascinated rather than exasperated me, so I became a clinician. When I tend to forget how much broader my understanding of human nature has grown, I have only to speak to friends who work in offices where they interact solely with their social peers. They remind me of my second-year student self, liberal in philosophy, aware of racial issues, but taking youth, absence of deformity, and life itself for granted. When I started clinical work my second year, it was quite a blow to learn that my social skills were as backward as my medical skills. I wanted to be useful, but I was in the way. I wanted to be liked and respected, but I was dismissed as young and female. I became more and more self-conscious.

My medicine rotation at the beginning of third year helped reverse many of these negative feelings. I worked at the county hospital, where simply the presence of another body was appreciated. The patients didn't expect Marcus Welby, and the ward team I joined asked as much of me as I could give. In retrospect, launching into a demanding clerkship was the best prescription that could have been written for the self-doubt of second year. Yet I remember crying when I reached home with my assignment. All the upper-class students had told me that the medicine clerkship was too important to take first and I had believed them.

Which leads to an important second-year job that I have not yet discussed: planning the next two years of study.

At all schools with which I am familiar there is considerable leeway in the organization of clerkships, the clinical specialty rotations that replace the classroom in the last two years. There are standard required clerkships such as internal medicine, pediatrics, obstetrics and gynecology, surgery, and perhaps ambulatory care or family medicine. There are electives like radiology, opthalmology, and the intensive care unit. Generally, the required clerkships must be largely finished in the third year, especially since, in many cases, they are prerequisites for electives. But in order to accommodate all the students on the wards in small groups, everyone at my school had to have a different schedule. In our class of 150, we submitted our choice of pathways and entered a computer lottery. Once the pathway was spit out with our names on it, there was no appeal. I imagine a smaller school would have more flexibility.

Are there any rules for choosing a pathway, given that they will necessarily vary from student to student? As usual, I think the best advice is, know thyself. Have you already chosen a field like anesthesia or pediatrics? Then you need to do that clerkship early on—to confirm your choice and to allow you the option of pursuing electives in that field before recommendations for internship are due, in the fall of the fourth year. Are you totally exhausted by the end of second year and in need of family time to rebuild your relationships? Take a month of vacation before you start spending thirty-six-hour days in the hospital. Are you unsure of what kind of doctor you want to be? Take a general clerkship like surgery or medicine early on to give you an overview of a large field. It is true that the recommendations from the long, required clerkships are important, but the staff recognizes the difference between a student at the beginning of the third year and the end, and judges him accordingly. For me, taking medicine early, my enthusiasm counted more and my ignorance less. I am also the kind of person who does best tackling the most stressful task first: If I wait, I have too much time to think myself into fear. Similarly, I would rather work hard for a while, then relax totally, than spread a task over a longer time. So I saved all my vacation time for the end and actually graduated in March of my last year, to have a true break before internship. You have to determine what pattern of study works best for you.

If you are anxious to be accepted in a particular internship program, you should try to do a clerkship in your field at that institution before the end of the first semester, fourth year, since programs choose interns early second semester. I should emphasize *in your field* because it is amazing how little communication there is between academic departments. The vascular surgery professor you impress may be a stranger to the pediatrics department or, worse yet, may be regarded as a buffoon. Obviously, if the head of the internship committee is a nephrologist and you choose a nephrology clerkship and do well, you have an advantage at selection time. I knew students who chose all their clerkships in this manner, but their strategy didn't always work.

Remember, also, that this will be your last opportunity to experiment outside your chosen field. My friends laughed at me for taking family practice and intensive care nursery since I intended to go into medicine, but I had plenty of opportunities to take the subspecialty clerkships such as pulmonary and cardiology as a resident and I never felt handicapped. If I had it to do over again, I would take more orthopedics, ear, nose, and throat, and gynecology: Every practicing internist needs some background in these fields.

Or better yet, I would spend the year abroad, as did some of my colleagues.

Certain residencies, such as psychiatry and ophthalmology, fill their places years in advance, so second year is the time to apply for a position. If you are interested in one of these fields you must do your program shopping early and find an adviser in your field to show you the ropes. If you decide later, you may have to work for a year after internship, for all the places may be filled.

The options may seem overwhelming. "How do I know what kind of doctor I want to be?" you moan. "I haven't even been on the wards yet." I agree it's a crazy system, geared to those who enter school knowing their subspecialty. Take comfort in the fact that people change their minds all along the way. It is common for interns to switch fields, even though they have to repeat part of their internship. And it is not unusual for residents who have completed three years of surgery or medicine to switch to radiology or anesthesia. At that point they are usually making life-style decisions, seeking better pay for fewer hours. As you begin your third year and start to make your own career decisions, watch how the doctors you admire live. Everyone appreciates the decisiveness and skill of the trauma surgeon, but how many of us want to be on call for the rest of our lives? While it is no tragedy to take extra training, a realistic assessment of family and career goals during the second year can save years of unnecessary toil.

At times I almost envied those in my class who were motivated solely by greed. No balancing of social conscience, family financial considerations, geographical preference for them. You should consider all these things as you plan your schedule for the last two years, but bear in mind that most of the doctors I have asked over the years tell me that their choice of field was an emotional rather than a rational decision. They admired a particular professor or enjoyed a clerkship they did not expect to like. I felt most at home in medicine, period.

At the end of the second year, there is one more hurdle to scale before hitting the wards: the first part of the three-part National Board Exam. Medical schools vary in the amount of weight they lend to this exam. Many use it as a final exam for the first two years, a prerequisite for starting clinical work. Some schools allow students several weeks to study for it; others expect them to take it in stride, along with the regular finals for the semester or quarter. At my school, rumor had it that the failure rate was 10 percent—high enough to worry. I do believe that it was the most difficult of the three tests.

So, study. My study group bought a set of books with questions similar to those on the exam and systematically worked our way through them, week by week. I remember how certain immunology questions would send us into peals of laughter, they seemed so hopelessly obscure. Fortunately, the test itself was not as bad as those questions, so we all passed. Incidentally, studying from the previous year's exams was a technique we used all through medical school with great success. It is a good way to find out what the instructor considers important and is ideal for a group situation, since generally someone will understand the answer provided, even if you don't.

If you don't pass the first time around and are allowed to proceed onto the wards anyway, think five or six times before deciding to forget the National Boards and, as some students I know did; instead take the FLEX at the end of medical school or internship. The sediment of the clinical years will soon bury the mountain of preclinical work, and digging down for that bedrock will be more difficult three years hence, when you are eligible for the FLEX, than one year ahead, when you will be able to retake Part I. Of course, if you plan to practice in one of the two states where only the FLEX is recognized, you have no choice. Just might make you think twice about moving to Louisiana or Texas, though.

5

THIRD YEAR: ON THE WARDS

Welcome to life in the fast lane. The third-year student starting out on the wards needs the concentration of a chess master, the speed of a sprinter, the balance of a skier, and the endurance of a marathon runner—all at once. Fatigue is like a muscle kink that won't go away, drawing you up short from time to time. And the family—well, the family just can't believe it. Lulled by the first two years, spouses feel they have adjusted pretty well until suddenly you're gone. "I wouldn't mind your studying all the time, if you would just come home," they moan over the phone. And you wonder who has the harder job, the student or the one at home alone.

This year represents a clean break from all previous classroom training. Since the transition requires quite a bit of adaptation, I have divided this chapter into two parts.

The first part is a general description of the clerkship experience, the second a brief description of specific rotations.

CLERKSHIP EXPERIENCE

The clerkship format sounds logical enough. In order to introduce the doctor-in-training to different fields while he learns basic clinical skills, he rotates from service to service in an acute-care hospital. The work is in the hospital because the concentration of pathology is denser and supervision can be closer than in an outpatient setting. Didactic sessions alternate with hands-on patient care on the ward, where the student is usually part of a team consisting of a hierarchy of students, interns, and residents. Interns and residents, who have graduated from medical school, are the "house officers" who actually care for the patient, supervised by an "attending" or "visit" who is a fully licensed physician and bears the legal responsibility. The third-year student finds himself clinging to the bottom of the ladder of clinical prowess. On morning rounds, when the team assesses the condition of the patients, the student fields medical questions from house staff and attending. "What are the complications of diabetes?" "What are the signs of a wound infection?" Later the student trails after the intern, learning practical skills like starting intravenous lines and serving as a general go-fer. There may be several hours of classroom work directed at the students or conferences that the entire staff attends. On most services, the student examines or "works up" a proportion of the cases that he must then present to the attending. Then, after such a typical day ends at five or six, the student takes call with his team. That is, he stays in the hospital overnight every other or every third or every fourth night to cover any emergencies that arise, and admit patients at night. He may or may not be able to sleep during the night, depending on the patient load. But the next day he must perform all his usual duties, regardless of whether he slept or not. In other words, he works a thirty-six-hour shift.

Of course, this routine varies from clerkship to clerkship, from hospital to hospital, from school to school. Most psychiatry clerkships do not require students to stay the night: Psychiatric emergencies are not central to psychiatric practice. Some schools feel that staying up all night is unnecessary at the third-year level, when learning to examine a patient is more important than crisis management. But even when night call is not required and even where sleeping facilities are not provided for third-year students, they may end up in the hospital at all hours.

Why do students stay if their presence is not formally required and loved ones are waiting? Well, it is exciting. After two years of rote memorization, here are real live patients who are sick, often very sick. Their status may be changing from hour to hour. The rest of the team is staying to care for them, agonizing over the diagnosis and the appropriate therapy. Maybe the intern will let the student assist during the lumbar puncture, or an extra hand may be needed to wheel the patient down for an emergency X ray. Or perhaps the student has never seen an appendectomy or the birth of twins. How can he just go home?

After a few sleepless nights, however, most students find that they can live without seeing every operation. After all, someone else will probably need an appendectomy in the daytime before the clerkship is over. Yet still he stays, for he has discovered the first universal rule of clerkships: It is important to study, but it is more important to be seen studying. Never mind that you have a newer edition of the same book at home, where you could read it at a desk and take notes in peace and quiet. Your resident won't see you reading it at home and you will not receive the same brownie points as your classmate huddled in the other corner of the room, apparently so deeply engrossed in the text that he has not noticed the intern flicking ashes on him.

It is contemptible and you are ashamed to admit even to yourself, but you are competing with all the other third-year students. You may not be the brightest or the most dexterous, but you can sure be the most enthusiastic. If you just push yourself a little harder, you can be the last to bed and the first up; you can make your cheerful presence indispensable to the team. Now, there is a mighty fine line between enthusiasm and apple-polishing, and your performance is subject to interpretation. But as they say in show business, exposure counts.

The principal showcase for your knowledge is the presentation. After second year, it is assumed that the student knows how to structure a presentation, but this is not always the case, particularly since the requirements change from clerkship to clerkship. Half the time professors seem to want the complete production just as it was taught second year, but the rest of the time they request a truncated version and grow impatient if the student gives the presentation as he learned it. As a rule of thumb, if the session is limited to third-year students, better prepare the authoritative version. But if the setting is ward rounds or another situation where people at various levels of the medical hierarchy participate, give short shrift to everything except the history of the present illness and pertinent positives or negatives in the past history. The reason for this change is that in the latter situation you are trying to convey information rather than perform an exercise, which was the case second year.

A Chinese resident taught me how to give a succinct

presentation. "First," he said, "sit across from or next to the attending." I immediately objected, "Won't that make me appear to be fawning over him?" He told me to think of it in terms of respect. No matter what I thought of the attending, I should respect his age and the achievement that his career represented. That Asian perspective pleased me and I listened as he continued, "Remember that the attending is a busy man, with a great deal on his mind. Don't waste his time. Give him a picture of the patient in the first sentence, to orient everything that is to follow." For instance, if a diabetic patient who has had a coronary bypass graft is admitted for a leg ulcer, say, "This is a forty-nine-year-old white man with a ten-year history of insulin-dependent diabetes, status post triple-vessel coronary artery bypass graft in 1979, who now presents with a nonhealing ulcer on his left great toe." After such a sentence, the attending can take a nap during the rest of the presentation and still discuss the case intelligently. Similarly, the presenter is off the hook, since even if he clutches and forgets the rest of his speech, he has included the essentials. Of course, the obstetrician will want to know the patient's parity in the first sentence, and the neurologist will expect you to mention whether the patient is right- or left-handed, but the principle is the same. Finally, my mentor suggested that I should organize the lab values by remembering to present first the results of those tests that a middle-aged attending would have been able to obtain overnight when he was a resident. That means the urinalysis and blood count always come first among the myriad chemistries that are now all too routine.

Some schools require that students memorize their presentations entirely; other permit note cards. While it is more impressive to speak from memory, even when not required, I think accuracy is more impressive than show-manship. You may well be repeatedly interrupted, so you must be able to pick up the story without starting all over. Avoid all unnecessary abbreviations and speak authoritatively. The exam you present is assumed to be your exam, so don't preface every finding with "I thought I heard" or "I thought I felt." Read the resident's workup before rounds and try to resolve any discrepancies between his findings and your own by returning to the bedside. If you still cannot hear the third heart sound, present his exam or your own—not both. Your conscience must be your guide. Never, but never, make up an exam. If you did not perform the pelvic, say, "The pelvic, as performed by the intern, was unremarkable." If the attending asks what the amylase was and you do not think an amylase was sent, say so. A cowardly resident will jump in at that point and say, "It is pending, sir." Let him do the lying, for it is his responsibility.

Most students (and physicians, for that matter) seriously underestimate the value of the history in making a diagnosis. Professors urge its importance but rarely take the time to demonstrate the technique. Especially nowadays, when patients can pass through total body scanners on their way from the emergency room to the ward, it is difficult to believe that anything the patient has to say matters. Listening to another human being also takes time, particularly if that person is uneducated or speaks a foreign language. As an internist, I often find that my role as a consultant is to use my relatively cheap time to listen to what the higher priced surgeon is too busy to hear. As a student, I once watched the chief surgical resident bellow "Dolor?" over and over again as he prodded a brown-skinned patient's abdomen. I knew he was not likely to elicit a verbal response, since the patient spoke Arabic and not Spanish, but I was too chicken to say so.

Once again, it was a resident who taught me how to obtain a reliable history, that is, one that the patient will not deny the next morning in front of the attending. Nothing is more demoralizing to the beleaguered student than to stand by and watch the story it took him two hours to obtain be contradicted. The trick is to repeat back to the patient all the crucial points. It is phenomenal how many times a man who has just finished telling you how he first started coughing the night before last will change his mind when you play it back in stronger terms: "Let's see, as I understand it, you were entirely well until the day before yesterday . . ." "Oh, no," he interrupts, "I've had a little cough for two or three weeks." And so forth. I warn you, the price for such accuracy is time, perhaps more than you are allowed or can spare. Don't kid yourself that the resident who whizzes in and out of the patient's room in ten minutes is getting the full story. He just has nine more patients to see before he sleeps. Speaking of time, always, but always, make sure the patient is with the program before you go for the gory details. It does not help to learn that he stopped drinking twenty years ago if he believes that it is 1945 and is not certain whether Roosevelt is still President.

Third-year students are considered fair game for any question, any time. And *game* is the word for some interrogations that are basically rhetorical: There are not many human beings who can cogently describe the fate of a chylomicron in the liver or compare the various regimens for adjuvant chemotherapy in the treatment of breast cancer off the top of their heads. If you have the time to read up on such topics, more power to you. But you will be held responsible for the classic clinical presentations and standard therapy for the diseases you encounter.

Which brings us to the second rule of the third year: Read the textbook first. Your well-meaning resident who is showering you with arcane references does not expect you to read them all. But if you admit a patient with pneumoccocal pneumonia you'd better remember to note whether his sputum was blood-streaked. And if you want to win friends and influence people, it is best to read the textbook before your presentation, in order to abstract the pathology he represents. It's like bird-watching: A photograph of an individual of a species may be more "realistic" than a generalized illustration emphasizing distinctive markings, but given the range of individual variation, twenty photographs might be required to teach the same pattern recognition that the illustration provides. The textbook is your illustration. Of course, patients can talk, which often confuses the issue. "Well, the pain started a few hours after I ate that crab salad sandwich, Doc," may introduce a case of food poisoning, but the patient may actually have appendicitis and the fact that he ate a sandwich turn out to be totally irrelevant. These false clues are the red herrings of medicine, and if the road to hell is paved with good intentions, the path to the wrong diagnosis reeks of fish.

When to do this reading? The wee hours of the morning may be the only time available, but it is tough to stay awake to read. When you are busy caring for patients, adrenaline is the only drug you can rely on. Caffeine and amphetamine render the abuser more wired than awake. And he or she ultimately crashes. As a medical student, you cannot afford either extreme. I never knew how sensitive I was to caffeine until I tried to start intravenous lines after two cups of coffee. A fine caffeine tremor would emerge that not only compromised my manual dexterity but signaled to the patient that I was nervous even if, as in later years, I wasn't. Those who study biological clocks tell us that body temperature dips at night. I found I had to bring a sweater for my nights on call. I also had to eat like a bird—nonstop. I would pack carrots and celery and cheese and crackers to keep myself from the vending machines, but I always ran out of my stash before the night was over and bought potato chips, too. Fortunately my metabolism is such that I did not gain weight: I lost ten pounds in the first two weeks of junior medicine. Terror is an effective method of weight control. If you absolutely cannot keep your eyes open to read, don't worry. Later on, when you have more responsibility, terror will keep you awake also.

Up to this point I have emphasized the interaction between the student and the attending because that performance is the stuff of which grades are fashioned. However, it is the house staff who do the bulk of the teaching and all of the patient care, legal niceties to the contrary. While it is easier to develop a friendly relationship with interns or residents since they are, after all, only a few years further along in their training, long hours of forced intimacy create problems of their own. The camaraderie of a well-functioning ward team is one of the delights of medical education. Like the little girl in the nursery rhyme, when it is good, it is very, very good, and when it is bad, it is horrid. Given the forced nature of the group, it could hardly be otherwise. Besides working all day with each other, typically sharing one or two meals, the members of the team also work all night, often sleeping in coed quarters. Since clerkships range in length from one to three months, there is no time to warm up to the group. In effect, the students, and to a lesser extent, the house staff, are required to change jobs every few months. And the whole process of starting a new job—anticipation, performance anxiety, proving competence, and making friends—is telescoped into hours or, at most, days. While there may be a few particularly self-confident, gregarious fellows to whom such constant change seems natural, on most stress lists, changing jobs ranks right up there with death in the family or moving.

There are tricks to ease these transitions, some of which students adopt in self-defense more than anything else. I think the most important of these is to try to keep your relationships superficial initially. You may well find that the less you know about your teammates' personal lives and political beliefs, the better. I remember that when I started the cancer service as an intern I was greeted by three white men: a fellow intern with a thick Southern accent, a resident with a Southern accent, and a fellow from South Africa. By that time I had learned to take a deep breath and say to myself, "We are all here to care for patients." And except for a few tense moments when the South African described the wonderful variety of pathology that tuberculosis produces among the "natives" of his country, we did very well. In fact, the Southern intern became my closest friend in the internship class.

So there are advantages to random rotation: You meet people you'd never have approached socially who end up deeply enriching your life. I know women who have dated a good proportion of their residents. And I have friends who met their spouses on a thirty-six-hour shift. Just remember, unlike an office, you can't leave your co-workers behind at five o'clock. For the same reason, it is incumbent upon you to be as discreet as possible with the confidences of others. It is amazing what topics of conversation emerge through the fog of fatigue. Suddenly an acquaintance of a few days will start talking about his operation for thyroid cancer or his mother's death after years of struggling with multiple sclerosis. Death is close in a hospital night and it helps to talk. But don't be surprised if the intern who was so open with you one lonely dawn doesn't speak to you when you rotate off service. It goes with the territory. I always suffered from resident withdrawal as a student and an intern, if I liked the resident. They seemed so competent and dynamic that I wondered if I could ever fill their shoes. Now I wonder, did I?

Unless you have the cool of the iceman, you will find there are people you absolutely hate and people you absolutely love. As a student, I found there were certain house staff members who viewed my presence as an intrusion into their space. They made no effort to teach but would send me on errands that seemed contrived to keep me from where the action was. Usually, there is another team member who is more helpful, but if not, it may be just tough luck. Two other rules of this year are, There is no appeal, and its corollary, The student is always wrong. As far as I can tell, these rules originated in team sports and the military. Why they should apply to the ward situation was never clear to me, but I assume it has to do with male bonding or some such mystery. At any rate, the ideal student is supposed to accept whatever inequities occur with a smile, even if he or she is treated capriciously or evaluated in a prejudicial manner. You put yourself in double jeopardy by complaining, for you will be labeled as having a bad attitude or not being a team player.

This is the point at which personality and poise count more than knowledge. The evaluations that matter are those of the attendings, with whom the student often has minimal contact and that contact only through the formal presentations. Sometimes the attending changes from week to week, so a judgment is based on a single presentation. In addition, students can be called upon to criticize one another's presentations and downgraded if they don't go for the jugular. "What does it make you feel like, to be shown up by a woman?" a male friend was asked after his partner's presentation. The competition is direct and fierce and in territory previously considered off-limits in the days of objective written work.

Like personal appearance. Many doctors feel it is entirely appropriate to comment on whether a man wears a beard or a woman, pants. I encountered a surgery professor who would not pass anyone who did not wear a tie. Snap assessments are the order of the day, and woe to the shy student. It is crucial that the first presentation to any attending be the best you can do, because that impression is the one that will stick. Women have to go out of their way to be assertive, since many professors' inclination is to assume that they are too frail to hang with the boys. I learned this lesson very well, because I went through medical school with a male control, my husband. On any written test, I would do as well or better than he, including the tests we took at the end of every clerkship. I also tend to talk more in classes, asking questions or offering answers. However, I was repeatedly criticized for being too quiet. It was obvious to both of us that no one was going to call a six-feet, three-inch black man nonassertive, even if he never opened his mouth. On the only clerkship we took on the same ward at the same time, he was recommended for honors but placed too low on the written test to receive them, whereas I, who received the second highest grade out of a class of 150 students, was not recommended for honors because I failed to make a strong enough impression. It is said that doctors like to create doctors in their own image, so the further you deviate from that image, the harder it is going to be. And my experience suggests that the opposite sex is perceived as more deviant than another race.

Granted, then, that you should know better than to complain, what can you reasonably expect from house staff? First, tolerance, as you tag along. A phenomenal amount of learning during these years occurs by osmosis: It is like the concept of total immersion in a foreign language. The conscientious student tries to shadow his patients and the intern at the same time. This is the time to find out what actually happens to the patient after a requisition for an echocardiogram is casually completed. Or, if the intern is delivering a baby or performing a bone marrow, the student should try to be there and, after a short while, to help. I do not mean to imply that the third year is the best time to learn to perform procedures, other than perhaps starting intravenous lines. As the professors will emphasize, internship is a whole year of procedures and the focus of the third-year student should remain on theory, not practice. But attacking a patient with a needle is an irresistible attraction to the neophyte on the ward, and it is also a chance to engage the house staff in conversation about indications for the test, cautions, complications. However, please don't initiate your questioning in front of the patient. Nobody wants to hear how many ways you can die from a required procedure, even if he was told of the possiblity of death when he signed the consent. I think it is natural, while the student is hanging around, for him to give the intern a hand: Fetch the scissors or open the needles. This sort of busywork is referred to as "scut" and is much disdained by house staff. However, it is my conviction that at the third-year level, scut in reasonable quantities can be a learning experience. It will endear you to the intern, who is unspeakably hassled, and is fair exchange for your questions. And students do tend to forget how much their presence slows the house staff, to whom time is of the essence. The good student rivals a two-year-old in tenacity, "But *why* do you do that?" There were times as a resident when I felt like a harried mother with four or five children clutching at my skirts. So go easy. Remember that your intern also has a family he'd like to see occasionally.

On the other hand, do not allow yourself to be exploited. There is no learning value for anyone in running to the cafeteria for coffee. If you want to do it, and I certainly have, fine. But the house staff should have the good grace to regard that as a favor, not as part of your duties. And don't forget your own obligations, which you must keep, even if it feels odd to leave the team for a lecture. If didactic sessions are scheduled for you, inform your resident and leave. Don't stay to help out "just this once" because the intern urges you to. A third-year student is neither fish nor fowl; he straddles the classroom and the ward. It is not easy to serve two taskmasters, so you must guard against overcommitment. If you know you have a class in the afternoon, don't agree to check the afternoon lab values just to please your resident. I assure you he will not be pleased if he expects the lab at four and your class doesn't end until six. The cardinal sin on the ward is to leave undone that which you ought to have done, particularly if it jeopardizes patient care or places an additional burden on one of your teammates.

In order to receive the most teaching, always express

interest in whatever field you are studying, because house staff and attendings alike tend to ignore the student who announces from the beginning that he has chosen a different specialty. I think that this is shortsighted of them—who needs to learn more surgery as a third-year student, the surgeon who will hear it all again or the internist for whom this is the last shot? Common sense notwithstanding, ego is ego, and everyone likes to think that his or her specialty is the finest. I never used to know what to say when a urologist would sarcastically ask, "I don't suppose you're going into urology?" (there are six board-certified women urologists in the country), but now I would answer, "I'm thinking about it." That's honest: At the time I *was* thinking about it—thinking how much I would hate it.

Unlike every other member of the ward team, the third-year student has extra time to sit and chat with patients and their families. Often he can best contribute to the medical effort by holding the patient's hand while others probe. He can serve as a translator for "explanations" delivered by the attending in straight medical jargon. And he can trouble-shoot by keeping an eye on the patient's day-to-day routine and serving as a liaison with the nurses, dieticians, and therapists. In fact, some patients rely so much on the student that they relate to him as the primary physician, knowing full well his student status. Thus flattered, the budding clinician finds the classroom exasperating. Don't neglect it, though, for there are no grades given for bedside manner.

Still, the relationships you develop with your patients will sustain you through all the other nonsense you have to face. "Learn from your patients," say the old clinicians. "You will remember these first ones better than any that come afterward." And they are right. Certain diseases immediately summon to mind the first person I know who had them. Myasthenia gravis recalls a retired piano teacher from a rural county who was in and out of the intensive care unit with respiratory failure but refused to move closer to the medical center. She was determined to die alone if necessary, without even the solace of her music because her hands were too weak to play.

The words *acute renal failure* summon up a retarded man who swore he had given a urine sample in the emergency room (which we never found) but who did not urinate for the subsequent two weeks. I remember the importance of daily weighings in the management of this condition because one day the nurse charted his weight as fifty pounds less than the previous day's measurement. When I asked her about the discrepancy in my mildest humble-student manner, she scowled, "Well, he didn't eat breakfast today, you know!" I remember the thirteen-year-old who had run away from home with her fourteen-year-old boy-friend when they learned she was pregnant: Her baby was the first premature infant I ever saw resuscitated. The list goes on and on.

This year is a golden opportunity to learn what living with a chronic disease means. Hospital training is by nature episodic: The patients come in and out; you rotate services. As a house officer, you will follow a few clinic patients over a longer term, but it will take you years to get to know them and their families as well as you can during afternoon conversations over a few weeks in the hospital. And, for once, not really being the doctor can be an advantage, for you don't wield the knife or bear the evil tidings.

I can write this easily now, but at the time, the few procedures that I did learn as a third-year student were tremendous sources of anxiety in my dealings with patients. Drawing blood and starting intravenous lines require a human being for practice. Each time I approached a patient with a needle, I had to squelch the intrusive thought that everyone else on the team was more skilled than I and that the patient would suffer from my inexperience. If I missed the first time, as I almost always did, I wanted to stop torturing the patient and call for help. Some patients, understandably, reinforced my insecurity by complaining, "Why don't you get a real doctor. Stop experimenting on me." At that point, I was generally close to tears. But if I didn't try again, how would I ever learn? So I made a rule, all through my training: three strikes and I was out. As the years passed, I became a whiz at starting i.v.s. But even as a third-year resident, if by some quirk I could not start the line, I would leave and try to find help, even from someone my junior. Failing that, I would just leave and return a half hour later, generally to meet with immediate success.

When I admitted defeat, I knew I would face an exasperated and sometimes scornful house officer. But that was easier for me than to make a pincushion out of someone. Other students would just keep trying, afraid to ask for help. Of all the macho excesses of medical training, I think the fear of asking for help is absolutely the worst, since the patient is the one who suffers. "See one, do one, teach one" might be a reasonable approach to some standardized mechanical process like shelling peas, but it should be drummed out of medical education. It creates totally unrealistic expectations of immediate competency. A very few people never learn to start an i.v. reliably, for, like most things, it is not as easy as it looks. I bet there is an optimal way to shell peas, too.

I remember seeing a friend who had been on vacation shortly after I started third-year medicine. He was tanned, but mostly I noticed what splendid pipelines he had for veins. Another friend, now a surgeon, who had little experience in medical school starting lines, dreamed of veins bleeding under the skin during his first rotation as an intern. Believe me, the process is intimidating for everyone. But one day your hands will do exactly as you command. I knew how far I had come when I managed to place an i.v. in an addict who had used up all his obvious veins. It took me two tries, as an intern, but I later learned that on a prior admission the patient had required surgery for venous access and that the senior resident had just sent me to try because he knew a "little girl" like me couldn't do it. A nurse who had overheard the resident making fun of me clued me in afterward. And they claim there is no such thing as female solidarity!

So far I have extolled the rewards of treating patients as people and warned that your grades will not reflect any expertise you develop in that area. In fact, you may well encounter criticism if you respond to a patient directly. At the end of a formal interview in front of a group of medical students and their psychiatrist teacher, a patient once asked a classmate if he was wearing Earth Shoes. (Remember them?) He answered yes, and said that they were indeed comfortable. The psychiatrist exploded after the patient left. To answer such a question was a serious abrogation of professional conduct. "Never, never let a patient ask you a question," the psychiatrist instructed. My classmate's reaction, typically, was, "What's the big deal?" When I first heard the story, I seriously debated the validity of the psychiatrist's assertion, which I now know reflected his Freudian training and was an inappropriate instruction for a class in general interviewing skills. If a therapeutic relationship outside of analysis is threatened by responding to such a totally innocent question, it is not much of a relationship.

On the other hand, I can offer little advice as to what constitutes an appropriate therapeutic stance. I do not advise you to be yourself. The women's movement notwithstanding, patients do not seek a friend in their physician. They seek someone they can respect and who will respect them. The problem is that trivial attributes influence what they think as much as your competence, which, after all, they are rarely in a position to judge. I don't wear jeans to the office, and I don't swear. I don't call my patients by their first names unless I would feel comfortable being so addressed. I do my darnedest to look older by wearing skirts and heels and makeup, and still field questions about my age (that is, competence) with every other new patient. How I envy my associate who is balding! Yet when I was eight months pregnant I could hardly pretend I hadn't noticed. I gave my due date when asked, and the picture of my son in my office is as much for my patients' benefit as mine. How would the psychiatrist who criticized my classmate for extolling the virtues of his Earth Shoes have dealt with a pregnancy?

The bottom line is that traditionally doctors have not had to cope with their own pregnancies. Maybe other doctors feel as comfortable in three-piece suits as I feel in jeans. Perhaps an authoritarian stance comes naturally to them. I have been admonished for acting too maternally toward my patients. Are male students criticized for acting too paternally? Probably not, since a traditional father is so much more distant than a traditional mother. But while I am willing to dress like an older women and curb my opinionated tongue, somewhere along the line I decided that I would not deny my legitimate concerns to please some arbitrary standard of indifference. I do care about my patients' parents and their children and their lives.

So do most doctors, in every field. In fact, I am constantly amazed how many caring people survive the brutality of medical training. It has occurred to me that patients have no conception of the ridiculous amount of time doctors can spend making a decision: talking themselves into an operation or a therapy. As a primary-care physician, I worry over each consultation and weigh my consultant's recommendation against my knowledge of the patient's lifestyle and tenacity. How much is enough? What is too much? And you will, too, especially while in training. You must find the strength within yourself to overcome the paralysis of anxiety, however, or you should not take care of patients. A doctor must learn to live with ambiguity, to make decisions based on less than total knowledge, to feel as comfortable with gray as with black and white. To accept that life has mysteries beyond our understanding, that death is an inexorable roll call. I think of the third-year student, a stranger, who once accosted me in the hall when I was a resident and wailed, "I've only had four patients and three of them have died." Even when death is expected, perhaps desired, it diminishes us. That, too, is part of doctoring, a part that never becomes easier to accept, no matter how familiar.

Just when such cosmic issues threaten to overwhelm you, the theater of the absurd of hospital life will provide a distraction, like pondering the etiquette of the coed sleep room. This was not much of an issue for me on junior medicine; in two months I never found the room. I was at the county hospital, so I was afraid to go looking in strange corridors well after midnight when I was finally ready to nap, and I never had sense enough to locate it during the day. Frankly, I was also afraid of finding it, since I would never have had the nerve to turn on the light or to grope over several beds for an empty one in the dark. So I slept sitting in a classroom, my head on the desk. I suppose that was even more dangerous, but I could read until I conked out and avoid disturbing anyone.

As a resident, older and sleepier, I overcame my squeamishness and bedded down where I was assigned. Everyone is usually so tired that the awkwardness of the situation is minimized. If you have access to scrub clothes, they are socially acceptable pajamas. If you don't, the question of how much clothing to remove arises. I could manage to sleep in everything but my support pantyhose, which I would remove in the bathroom. I have a friend who can't sleep with his pants on and who was chewed out by a woman who objected to his appearing in front of her in Jockey shorts. Amy Vanderbilt does not address this situation. Standing in, I would arbitrate that he should have made every effort to avoid displaying himself and she should have ignored what she saw. As a student, you will not have to respond to emergencies, but consider trying to learn to sleep with more clothes on if you would be embarrassed to show up without them. There was a woman in our class, my husband tells me, who changed into a nightgown every night. And I have heard of a famous pediatric resuscitation during which the resident's breasts were swinging in and out of her gown as she pumped on the child's chest. At the other extreme is a friend with whom I once shared a room who slept with all his clothes on, on top of the covers, on his back. I worried about the discomfort my presence was creating for him until another friend assured me that he slept that way with him also. Perhaps someday women in medicine will be taken for granted, so architects will plan hospitals with sleep rooms for both sexes, but until then modesty is the best policy.

SPECIFIC ROTATIONS

At my medical school, there were eight required clerkships: three months of surgery, two months of medicine, six weeks each of pediatrics and obstetrics and gynecology, one month of neurology, one month of psychiatry, two months of ambulatory and community medicine, and two weeks of anesthesia. The amount of time awarded each department roughly corresponds with the status of that specialty, since each department is always lobbying for more time to teach what it considers the most important subject in the curriculum. For instance, most schools don't require anesthesia at all; the fact that we took even two weeks of it reflects our strong department. Surgery was considered so important that the three months were split into a two-month didactic junior clerkship and a one-month senior clerkship on the wards.

Most medical schools are affiliated with more than one teaching hospital, so clerkship experiences can vary widely. Just as prisons range from country clubs to snakepits, hospitals run the gamut from private spas to just a cut above the county jail. Many students, if given a choice, select the plush facility, seeking the easy way out. While it is true that such luxuries as competent, English-speaking nurses and therapists, intravenous teams, and phlebotomy teams facilitate patient care, I don't think that a private hospital is the best milieu for the serious student. Until you can draw blood from a turnip, you have no business delegating that task to someone else.

Some students choose the university or private hospital

because the attending staff is world-famous, or because the ratio of faculty to students is so high. Well, don't kid yourself. Those professors are not hanging out at the nurses' stations anxious to chew the fat. They are holed up in their labs except for the one month the department requires their presence on the ward, when they emerge, blinking in the clinical spotlight. With serendipitous exception, they dislike the cases at hand. This is a particular problem in medicine, where because of the proliferation of subspecialists, more often than not the senior residents are the best general internists in the hospital.

Surgeons are mercifully more pragmatic in outlook; they don't like to jawbone, they like to cut. Unfortunately, they are so much more invested in their hierarchy that the surgical attendings are as aloof as any internists. Surgical teams are run in a paramilitary fashion; the only response to the command "Jump!" is "How high?"

In view of these facts of life, I would rarely choose a clerkship by the reputation of the professors, unless I heard that one was truly awful. If you are able to choose a resident, that might be worthwhile, but since everyone rotates, it is rarely possible to intersect orbits. So choose the hospital with the largest accessible patient population. Third World students almost always feel more comfortable in a racially mixed situation. While I know of only isolated examples of patients refusing a doctor because of his color or sex, it is quite an ego boost to be doubly appreciated because of racial pride. I have heard of black patients giving more detailed histories to black students so that they could outshine their white classmates. It also stands to reason that a county hospital patient who is truly ill will be less fussy about his doctor's skin color than the executive admitted for a physical. Along the same lines, as a woman,

I would not choose a veterans' hospital for extended periods of time. Older men, the bulk of the veteran population, are perhaps the population group least receptive to the idea of women in medicine to begin with. Add to this the sexist tendencies of any men in a pack and you can have real trouble.

When I was an intern, a veteran with angina used to bait me so mercilessly on rounds that my resident turned to me as we walked away and admitted that he had never before realized how difficult it could be for women. Naturally, this patient who was so skeptical of my abilities chose the day my resident had a dentist's appointment to have a heart attack on the ward. It was lunchtime, and I had to start an i.v., scare up a nurse to get him nitroglycerin and morphine, and negotiate the bureaucracy to move him to the coronary care unit—all without leaving him unattended for more than a few seconds at a time. When he was safely in the unit, pain-free, he apologized to me for his previous behavior. I thought that was bloody decent of him, but it didn't make it all worthwhile.

On the other hand, there are those who want to avoid the sort of verbal and sometimes physical abuse common at the county hospital. Combative, intoxicated patients take some getting used to, but I preferred such straightforward interaction to the tiresome carping of the more pampered. I just tried to think of "motherfucker" as a term of endearment. If your school has comprehensive tests at the end of each clerkship, as mine did, you will be slightly handicapped by working in a county facility, where the range of diseases is usually not as broad as in the referral facility. However, I studied for the junior medicine test with my women's group, and though among us we had experience in every hospital setting our school offered, none of us found the questions on the previous year's test a piece of cake.

I offer my opinions about various kinds of hospitals because I learned the hard way, but I would advise you to try all the hospitals available to you at least once and make up your own mind. It will be helpful to be familiar with several systems when it comes time to choose an internship, and just moving from hospital to hospital helps shake academic dogmatism.

It is not easy for me to write about individual clerkships without betraying my extraordinary bias in favor of internal medicine. In retrospect, however, I can see how much of that bias was circumstantial. Perhaps if I had chosen my clerkships more with an eye to my own personality than to the "best" place via the grapevine, I would have been equally seduced by another field. I once met a radiologist who told me that her first love was internal medicine but that the brutal hours of her prestigious internship had driven her out of the field. Had she opted for less prestige, she might have made it as an internist. Clinical training is a long haul and clerkships are merely the warmup to postgraduate work. Don't exhaust yourself flexing your muscles.

One clerkship that should not exhaust anyone is psychiatry. It was glorious to have a nine-to-five job. I observed group and individual therapy and posed as a therapist myself to two patients whom I saw twice a week. Nothing I did in medical school made me as uncomfortable as playing therapist. Some poor guy who had called the crisis-intervention center was triaged to me, a student with no therapeutic training who would be rotating off service in a month. Psychiatrists are sensitive to teasing from their medical colleagues that they don't "do anything," but if they can set up third-year students as therapists, even under supervision, even they must not value their training much. On no other third-year clerkship was I identified as the primary-care provider.

I don't suppose the patients suffer irreparable harm from a parade of students, but our training was not very pertinent to the majority of us who did not become psychiatrists. There are estimates that up to 50 percent of patients who seek care from a primary-care practitioner have a significant functional, that is, nonorganic, component to their illness, but either by culture or personality these people are not usually amenable to traditional therapy. Doctors need help developing a therapeutic stance that can serve them in their day-to-day work, not a few weeks practice of a subtle art they are not likely to attempt again. The most valuable day of the course was a field trip to a state psychiatric hospital and a hospital for the mentally retarded. Every self-absorbed neurotic should have the opportunity to meet some true crazies. Society's motto is Out of sight, out of mind, and we leave psychiatrists holding the bag.

If psychiatry was a disappointment, obstetrics and gynecology was a revelation. Our rotation was divided into two three-week blocks: one for inpatient obstetrics—delivering babies—and one for outpatient obstetrics and gynecology and gynecological surgery. I chose to take the clerkship at the university hospital, because it was the one with the largest volume of deliveries. What I didn't fully appreciate when I made that decision was that the best obstetrical patients for students are low-risk multiparous women, who tend to be scarce at a teaching center. My husband at the county delivered fewer babies than I did, but the labors he attended were shorter and less agonizing than those of the first-time mothers I saw. Now I realize too that much of my reaction to the obstetrical ward was totally unprofessional. I would sit with a woman screaming for pain medicine and think, *This will be me someday*.

As usual, the third-year student role was ambiguous. Unlike the rest of the staff, who had other duties, we were supposed to stick with one woman until delivery. I would stare at the woman and her husband, who were too polite to ask me to leave but did their best to ignore me. After the long vigil, if there were no problems, I could assist in the delivery, which was a relief to all concerned. And joyous, except once, when a Chinese father rejected his little girl, refusing to hold her because she was not the son tradition mandated.

It seemed so hard. The female blood smell nauseated me, like breathing tampons. The inexorable contractions were terrible to watch, hour after hour. I hated the natural childbirth teachers who lied to women about pain. One mother who made it through the process with only one shot of Demerol berated herself for having a bad attitude. Her Lamaze teacher had told her that the pain was all mental, so she felt she had failed by noticing it. Not to speak of the women who "failed" by requiring anesthesia or a Caesarean section. They tried so hard to create a peak experience out of labor that they almost missed the point—the baby.

I began to understand why many obstetricians treat women like children. The women they see most often are reduced by pain to a childlike dependency. It is tough to be assertive when a contraction is tearing you apart and everyone in the hospital seems to feel free to violate you with pelvic examinations. Obstetricians must develop a benevolent, reassuring presence to cajole women through to delivery. It is not surprising, then, that some of them cross over the fine line into paternalism.

The only time I came close to fainting in medical school was observing a predawn Caesarean section. It was a combination of fatigue and no breakfast, not the operation, but it reinforced my growing conviction that obstetrics would not be my field. Caring for two patients in one body is tough. I sympathize with the feminists who want to goad practitioners into greater responsiveness to their adult patients, but I have also felt the interventionist urgency for the life of the child that prompts technological excesses.

Outpatient obstetrics was a typical clinic experience: I saw patients once, for belly checks. It's too bad human gestation couldn't be shortened to four weeks for teaching purposes. There is no sense of the rhythm of pregnancy in a one-spot visit, even seeing women at various stages. From the time the patient starts to show until term, the office visit is pretty standardized: record weight, check urine, monitor fetal heart tones. It bored me as a student and later it bored me as a patient.

Gynecology was more exciting: pelvic infections, looking under the microscope at vaginal discharges, feeling for lumps and bumps. Birth control counseling is never dull, since every woman's assessment of the options is different. Being a woman, I felt I had a definite edge, partly because I had learned to do a pelvic exam during a mutual exam session the women in our class had arranged at a women's alternative clinic. The men had learned on a rubber model. I also wasn't afraid of the patients. I have noticed most internists shy away from pelvics, although it is certainly part of our job. One colleague frequently quotes his gynecology professor, who told him that his exam was so inadequate that he would learn as much sticking his hand out the window as into a patient.

It's lucky I like gynecology, because women assume I

have expertise in the area just because of my sex. So every day I still use the gynecology I learned. Often I think of the resident who hustled me out of the exam room after watching my laborious pelvic on a massively obese woman. I was sure he was going to berate me for taking so long, but I couldn't feel her pelvic organs through her fat. Instead, he burst out laughing.

"I couldn't stand it," he sputtered. "Did you feel anything?"

"No," I admitted.

"Of course not. She's too damn fat. You don't need to try so hard next time."

The introduction to gynecology also included some long hours watching gynecologists remove women's reproductive organs. There is an operation called a pelvic exenteration, performed for advanced cervical cancer, in which everything goes—the ovaries, the uterus, the vagina, the rectum, the bladder. It ain't all delivering babies.

Pediatrics at the county hospital came as close to my expectations as any clerkship. Four weeks of outpatient clinic and two weeks of ward passed quickly. Pediatricians are the sweethearts of medicine, and kids aren't bad either. Sick children are not as much fun as well children, however. Fretful squish faces outnumbered playful moppets. Drop-in clinic was always exciting, since children are so inventive at harming themselves, but my favorite was well-baby clinic. The chief pediatrician was a tall patrician gentleman, silver-haired and as sensible as overshoes. He presided over the multiethnic chaos like an enlightened missionary, encouraging the adolescent mothers and without translation communicating approval to all. Whether Vietnamese, Laotian, Samoan, Filipina, Chicana, Chinese, black, or white, each mother's face shone with the same proud, shy look as she displayed her latest. In my mid-twenties, I was older than most of the women, but their motherhood awed me. To me, a baby was the ultimate adult responsibility. To them, a baby was what happened nine months after sex.

There were some evening clinics, but basically the routine was nine-to-five for the outpatient work. Night call was not required on the pediatric ward either, but the hotshots managed to spend nights in the hospital, so all of us had to stay late to compete. There were quite a few trauma patients: broken bones and heads. Rounding on them was tolerable because children are so resilient that they bounce back from accidents that would incapacitate an adult. The kids with chronic diseases were the heartbreakers. One of my patients was a nine-year-old with sickle-cell anemia, recovering from her latest stroke. She was paralyzed on one side and unable to talk.

Since it was the county hospital, we also had more than our share of child-abuse cases, which were tough on the staff as well as the kids. It was difficult for me to remain dispassionate as I approached a man who had slapped his baby around. Pediatricians always deal with the child's social milieu, since they are concerned with development. Other doctors could learn quite a bit from their approach. Even physical development doesn't necessarily stop in adolescence.

Many students find that there is one junior clerkship that just doesn't work out. Surgery was that clerkship for me. I had done well in medicine, my first ward experience, so I sailed in thinking that this clerkship business was not as hard as I'd feared. Well, surgery took the wind out of my sails. Instead of participating in a ward team, it was back to working up patients for show, like a second-year student. Talking to friends at other medical schools, I found that our surgery clerkship may be unique in that it is almost totally didactic—no patient care, no time in the operating room. What most students elsewhere do third year was reserved for fourth year, during another month of required senior surgery. We spent the two months of junior year examining patients already on the ward, who had often already had their operations. We presented the cases to private doctors who came in especially to listen to us. These outside attendings changed each week, so each presentation was a do-or-die performance. I remember some of the sessions lasting two hours, just for two cases. We were constantly interrupted to correct wording or form, and we were criticized for every comma. In retrospect, I find it ironic that the surgeons felt compelled to teach in this manner, since they are notorious for the shortest, least comprehensive exams of any doctors.

It was a definite demotion after the heady clinical whirl of medicine. Even the subspecialty lectures were boring. An elderly ophthalmologist droned on for three hours Friday mornings in a room darkened for slides as everyone struggled to keep awake. We toured eye clinic and ear, nose, and throat clinic but didn't learn to use a slit lamp or a head mirror, the tools of those trades. Some students started skipping lectures, but I plugged on. In conversations with my friends, I made no secret of the fact that I was unhappy, but I attended every class and received no grade lower than a B on my written work.

So after four weeks, it came as something of a shock to learn that the chief of surgery was planning to flunk me. After haranguing me for an hour or so, mostly about my attitude, which I knew was not unique, he told me he was going to recommend that my partner and I drop the clerkship halfway and repeat it at another hospital. When pressed, he admitted that he could tell I had a bad attitude from my first presentation, when I had failed to smile. I can't imagine why I didn't smile, since he had just finished chewing out a fellow student in a speech that started with a sentence that will always stand in my memory: "Well, if a C is the lowest grade, that presentation is an F."

The news that I was flunking floored me, but I squeaked out that I was not a quitter and that I would rather try to salvage the eight weeks. What I really meant was that twelve weeks of junior surgery would have been intolerable. Either I finished in eight weeks, or surgery would finish me. My partner, the student with whom I was paired for presentations, had a healthy reaction to the news of our failure. "The guy's psychotic," he exploded. We sat down and plotted our strategy, which was basically to work our tails off and smile more. I was lucky to have a partner who assumed we would work as a team. When asked to judge each other's presentations, we presented a solid front of mutual support, rather than go for the jugular as we were encouraged to do. We made it, together. When the chief announced at the exam following the clerkship that we would be grateful to him in five years, we exchanged the last of many sympathetic glances.

Five years later, not only am I not grateful, but I am still bitter. That martinet ruined surgery for me, of course, but he also tainted the rest of my clinical work. From then on I was wary and tight, assuming that professors were out to get me, no matter how smoothly the clerkship seemed to be going. I lost my innocence: The ordeal transformed me from a fresh, eager student to a cynical sycophant. The therapist I finally saw much later compared his gratuitous attack to a rape, since he had all the power and I had no appeal. I don't think I would have been a surgeon anyway, but I would have liked the chance to find out.

After my third-year experience, I did not approach senior surgery with an open mind. During that clerkship, we followed our patients to the operating room, scrubbed, and assisted. We belonged to a ward team and cared for patients pre-op and post-op. It was a useful experience. I worked with pleasant surgeons, and I think it might even have been fun if I hadn't been so terrified. It wasn't easy for anyone, though. One of my friends who was courted by the surgery department and seriously considered making a career of it described her last day in the operating room. She'd been up all night and holding retractors most of the day, fighting to stay awake, when one of the surgeons asked her the name of the vessel he was dissecting out. She blanked, and one big fat tear plopped right in the middle of the sterile field, into the patient's body. She still operates, but as a pathologist.

I took neurology just as computerized axial tomography, or CAT scans, special detailed brain X rays, were coming into general use. As one neurologist commented, they took all the fun out of neurology. When a patient appeared with a neurological deficiency, the game used to be to guess what part of the brain was affected. Now the CAT scan shows the lesion as clearly as a broken bone on an X ray. Neurologists are still strong on speculation, however. The clerkship was like medicine played at a slower speed. More discussion, less action. Depressing, too. Strokes, brain tumors, multiple sclerosis.

Anesthesia is accurately described as five minutes of terror (the induction) and five hours of boredom (monitoring the patient during the operation). I was intrigued to find that this was a field that women had pioneered, as nurse anesthetists. Two weeks was just enough time to observe several kinds of operations and learn the principles of intubation. I would have required much more practice to feel confident I could pass a breathing tube into the trachea in an emergency. During the lulls between blood pressure readings, I found myself studying the sociology of the operating room crew, which I had been too frightened to do on surgery. Seen as a monarchy, the surgeon is king, the nurses are servants, and the anesthesiologist is like a prime minister. His opinions are respected, his services are crucial, but he has to tolerate the king's whims.

Ambulatory and community medicine was a failed experiment in relevance. The idea was to provide an adult outpatient experience, with emphasis on the whole patient. Unsuspecting new patients were subjected to a three-hour interrogation and exam by a team consisting of a medical student, a pharmacy student, a nursing student, and sometimes a dietician intern. This awkward interview resembled a press conference more than a physician visit. Each specialty had its own ax to grind, and everyone resented the medical student. I came close to abandoning the patient to my anxious colleagues several times. During the fourth hour of the patient's visit, we would (in chorus) present the case to an outside attending. Therapy was instituted in his name, and the patient would return for follow-up to see me alone. I spent most of the follow-up visits trying to undo the harm of the first encounter. I think there is a place for professionals other than the physician in patient care, just not in the same room.

One day a week, we pursued special projects. I chose to learn about occupational medicine, so every Thursday I would join a small group of students on a field trip to a factory or other workplace. This minicourse was one of the highlights of medical school. Intimate, relevant, exciting—everything the rest of ambulatory medicine wasn't. If I had been more of a political animal, I would have chosen occupational medicine over internal medicine for my career.

Finally, medicine. As third-year students, we were incorporated into the ward team for better or for worse. From ward rounds at eight A.M., through the nights on call I shadowed my intern, learning patient care from the emergency room to discharge. With the cushion of the intern and the resident behind me, I knew I wasn't ultimately responsible for anything, but I took my work to heart. Our team was busy and I tried to learn everything, since everything was bewildering. It seemed as though I must have attended the wrong classes the first two years; half the time, not even the language was familiar. Every other question out of my mouth was, "So what is normal?" as test result after test result accumulated. How big was an enlarged heart or a normal liver? When I asked how big a normal testicle was, my instructor, a woman, laughed and passed on what she had been taught: to put a hand in someone's pants pocket and compare. Somehow she had never found that method useful.

There were times of frustration. A sense of inadequacy haunted me. Some of the patients treated me as a joke. When I wasn't all thumbs, I was in everyone's way. The reason the experience was positive overall was that every day I had the opportunity to show up at my workplace, drink coffee, joke with my co-workers, and work, instead of sit on my can all day listening to lectures. This fit with my image of an adult and a doctor, both roles I was desperate to assume. One particularly busy night, my resident and intern, off admitting patients, had to leave me to follow a diabetic in ketoacidosis (a life-threatening metabolic crisis caused by high blood sugar and no insulin). He was a nineteen-year-old junkie from the jail ward who had used all his peripheral veins shooting dope. My resident, who was the first person to tell me that a doctor didn't have to be a genius, just compulsive, instructed me to draw his blood every hour from a groin vein (which I had never done before) and test it for glucose and potassium on a machine I had never previously used. Each hour I called him with the results so he could change the insulin and intravenous fluid orders, based on the new values. By morning, I could not see straight, but the patient was out of danger and I felt I had made a contribution to his recovery. It was a heady feeling: I was hooked.

This has been a long chapter, but third year is a long year. I had always assumed that internship would be the worst year of my training, but third year won that distinction. Part of the problem was that my expectations were too high. I had thought that after the tedium of the first two years I would gracefully emerge as a mature clinician. And looking ahead to the tremendous number of hours an intern works awed me. An intern's role is clearly defined, however, if not glorious. There is relative job security if you are already accepted to a residency, since only gross negligence or indiscretion will precipitate your dismissal. You're not expected to be cheerful or attractive or interested or even particularly competent. You're just the intern slogging through, following orders and watching a new class of students perform.

6

THE
REAL WORLD
REVISITED

At a recent birthday party, I caught up with a college classmate I had not seen in at least five years. He had taken time off to do political work but ended up in medical school; he was a third-year student during my first year of private practice. It was a congenial, mixed (medical and nonmedical) gathering. Everyone had a few drinks and talked about old times. We talked some medicine, nothing serious, until rather abruptly James began to tell us about his first day on junior medicine. His ward team was rounding on a young woman with lupus erythematosus, a relatively uncommon disease of young, especially black, women, that involves the production of antibodies against the body's own genetic material. Since this material is found in every cell, every organ system can be affected, typically lungs, kidneys, joints, and sometimes the brain. Lucky patients have very mild disease, requiring little therapy, but in other patients, lupus behaves like a malignancy, ravaging organ after organ.

The patient James saw that morning was one of the unfortunate ones, and the discussion on rounds centered around whether her brain was affected, which is always a point of contention since there are no objective criteria to diagnose lupus cerebritis. According to James, the large team was deep in discussion at the bedside when the patient began to scream, "You don't care about me at all. You don't care how I feel or if I live or die. I'm just a case you're experimenting on." And on and on. The team started to back out of the room, using this outburst as further proof of her irrationality and probable brain involvement. No one addressed the patient. At this point, the physicians listening to the story knew what was coming. My friend's voice became more urgent. "They just walked out. They completely ignored her. I just stood there. I couldn't move. I mean, I *could not move*. I didn't know what to say. What did I know? But I started to think, hey, man. Maybe I'm not cut out for this job. How can I do this? How can I deal with this? And I just stood there."

By this time, the intensity of James's speech had stopped the party cold. We were all a little embarrassed. Should we respond to his tone of voice and turn the party into a medical rap group? While we were making up our minds, James recovered with an offhand joke about inexperience and the conversation moved on. We did James a disservice by ignoring his anecdote, though. It was a classic example of the third-year cry for affirmation. He wanted to hear from us that he was okay, that his response to the patient was normal, that the team was as insensitive as he perceived them. Of course, even telling the story, he did not dare presume that the team was wrong. He asked us what was wrong with him; he wondered whether he was unfit for his chosen profession. After all, everyone else seemed satisfied with the encounter. Either he was crazy or they were. And it couldn't be them.

Well, I'm here to tell you it can be them. It has taken five years of clinical experience for me to have the confidence to say that. I too used to believe that there was something wrong with me when I thought doctors were rude or insensitive. They told me I would get over it, to wait until I had more experience under my belt. I never did get entirely over it, though, and each time I hear that third-year student outburst, I feel the same hopeless mixture of anger and impotence all over again. "Did you ever think of quitting medicine?" one of my best junior students asked me as a senior resident. I looked her straight in the eye and answered truthfully, "Every day."

For many of us, third year represented the first encounter with fundamental self-doubt. Depression the first years we could explain away, for memorizing biochemistry was clearly light years away from clinical medicine. Once on the wards, however, depression seemed more significant. It had to mean something if we didn't immediately fit in. We started to measure ourselves against the interns and residents who seemed so sure of themselves, or against the professors who appeared truly omniscient at times. During the long hours in the hospital, we wondered how it could be that book-learning left us so helpless in front of a sick human being. And, all of a sudden, our support group was gone. Even the most unfriendly medical school class harbors a few kindred souls, whom we had managed to ferret out over the first two years. I sat with the same group of people day in and day out the second year, sharing gallows humor as well as notes. I drew none of them on my rotations, however—only absentminded academic types or intense young men scrambling to get ahead.

What has been an all-too-shared experience becomes an individual apprenticeship overnight. Comparing notes, even with close friends, is hampered by problems of translation, for the routine of each hospital, each clerkship, is different. "What's medicine like?" your buddy on psychiatry asks, a little fearfully, while you stand in awe of another friend who has already delivered three babies. Sure, you can go home and talk to your spouse, but so much happens each day that you cannot keep abreast. So you tell about Mr. Ryan's operation and not Mrs. Hughes's death, or you lament that you blew a presentation but don't get a chance to describe what grand rounds was about. Anyway, you're exhausted. Lots of times you barely get through dinner before you crash.

Hence the tendency for third-year students like James to behave inappropriately at social gatherings. At school, your defenses are up. At home, you're mostly too tired for analysis. But, day by day, the experiences accumulate and you ruminate. After a glass of wine, among old friends, you find yourself blurting out stories you never intended to tell. I remember that one evening my husband and I had finally managed to plan ahead enough to make a dinner date with some nonmedical friends. I was looking forward to a relaxing meal with a couple whose company I had missed. I wanted to pretend for the evening that I had a job like pushing papers. Well, I relaxed. So much so that when I started to describe what I was doing, in response to a question, I began to cry. I know they must have thought I was perfectly crazy to break down in the middle of a restaurant in response to some innocent query like "So what do you do in the hospital?" But it was the first time in several weeks that someone who cared about me, other than my long-suffering spouse, had addressed a question to me as a person rather than as a medical student. It was such a relief to realize that I could still analyze my experiences and that there were people in the world who valued my analysis, who wouldn't dismiss it out of hand as neurotic or irrelevant.

Most spouses understandably find such outbursts disconcerting. They start to view medical school as an uncontrollable germ infecting all aspects of life, and they can't understand why the student doesn't develop immunity after a while. The more the student tries to explain his life, the more it frustrates the roommate who yearns to speak of anything else. Yet channels of communication must remain open, or the student who is metamorphosing into a doctor will quickly become a stranger. "They can never understand what it is like," I have heard friends say of their wives. In some absolute sense, that's probably correct, just as no one can understand what it's like to have cancer or be blind.

Pragmatically, however, that sentence is always a cop-out. Sure, no one can ever experience another person's life. As I have amply described, even with both members of a couple in medical training, there is room for misunderstanding and profoundly separate perceptions. A strong commitment will bridge the gap enough to allow a relationship to survive, but it requires incredible feats of mutual tolerance—tolerance that includes allowing the student to ventilate in any terms he chooses. I have been close to slugging wives who simper, "Oh, how can you call a patient a turkey?" or "You shouldn't joke about a patient dying." Believe me, the only way to keep from exploding after dealing with an irrational patient who is thwarting every therapeutic gesture or after watching a terminal patient suffer day after day is to try to find the humor in the situation. If you don't want doctors to act like gods, then you have to allow them to be human, at least at home. Otherwise, couples just grow apart. The ultimate breakup may not occur until after clinical training is over, when the couple finally has enough time together to realize they don't know each other anymore. But it all starts third year.

My own experience suggests that the first four years of clinical training, third year through first-year residency, are a lousy time to make any stressful changes in real life. The tremendous insecurity of this period bullies students into seeking refuge in fixed relationships. Dating is so difficult, life is so difficult, that men who previously enjoyed the singles game suddenly want to settle down. It is too depressing to come home to an empty apartment. I say "men" because they can generally marry at will if they are so motivated; women medical students are not so overwhelmingly attractive. But the same psychology applies.

There are worse reasons for marriage, but there are certainly better ones. While it may seem convenient to have a partner on hold for the next few years, it is not an ideal way to build a relationship. One student in our class married and divorced in the same year, unable to sustain the momentum of his marriage through one senior medical clerkship. While that is extreme, I think most of us had thoughts of separating at some point during our early clinical years. As one spouse put it, "If this doesn't improve when David gets out, I'm leaving. I didn't marry to sit at home alone."

Of course, there are long-term relationships in which marriage is precipitated by the prospect of a move at the end of fourth year. I would offer better odds on those, since the couple had some time to get to know each other in less pressured times. Making the acquaintance of a clinical student or a house officer is like sizing up a deciduous tree in the winter: Without the foliage, you can't judge the shade it will cast.

In these days of cohabitation, the timing of the marriage ceremony is often of no great concern, postponable until both partners are ready for a more public commitment. My medical school extended invitations to official functions to the student and his or her significant other. Unfortunately for many older women, childbirth cannot be so conveniently deferred, especially if a thirty-year-old woman is contemplating subspecialty training—five years after medical school is minimum. The first few years in practice are not the ideal time to start a family either, so the fourth year may seem to be now or never. Some men don't relish the idea of starting a family at forty, either. So although I have some fairly fierce reservations about the effect on a child of having a mother or father who's an intern, I must admit that fourth year is the logical time to plan a child for many couples.

Senior year of medical school resembles senior year of high school, and senior year of college: a slack time that doesn't much count once requirements are finished and applications for internship completed. In addition, internship is slavery—but salaried—so a child would not have to be supported by school loans for long. So if a pregnancy can be planned for the end of third year, with a due date near the beginning or middle of fourth year, the baby should have the benefits of two parents until the internship starts. I need to point out, however, even to medical students, that conception and pregnancy are not among life's predictable events. Well-educated couples often assume that once the diaphragm is on the shelf, conception is automatic. A fertile couple is one that conceives within a year, not during the first cycle. It is axiomatic that physicians and their relatives will have more complications in any medical situation than controls, which may explain why virtually every woman I know over thirty has either had difficulty conceiving, or has miscarried, or has an ectopic pregnancy, but these misfortunes also befall the general population, albeit in lower frequency. Mother Nature just doesn't produce on demand. This is less of a problem for medical student fathers, since they will not run the risk of waddling into their internship in their eighth month, but they will not have much time to spend with the baby. The story of a friend in my internship class is typical: In order for Sam to be with his wife at the birth, another intern had to work two nights in a row. When it was time for Sandy to come home from the hospital, he was on call again, so her mother brought her home. Actually, most of the women I know who had babies while in medical school ended up taking longer to finish. Since medical school is in session year round and clerkships only last a couple of months, you can take as much or as little time as your dean will allow.

Remember also that pregnancy is not necessarily a blissful physical experience. I was sick for the first five months, and believe me, the smells of a hospital are not what the doctor ordered for morning sickness. In private practice, I could discreetly vomit between patients. Had I been a resident, I might have found myself vomiting in the elevator, as did one superwoman I know who became pregnant during her internship. Another friend who had severe leg swellings during her first pregnancy attributes the problem to having been an intern, since a subsequent pregnancy was without incident. Finally, there is the psychological trauma of putting your sexuality out front (pun intended). I coped as best I could with my colleagues in training by trying to be one of the boys. There were guys in my residency group that I felt as close to as any men I have ever known, but we didn't discuss my menstrual cramps. Pregnancy is like a red F for *female*, which glares down any hope of being just another doctor like neon through fog.

One surgeon expecting his second child told me that he didn't remember being up much with his first baby; his wife reminded him that he was an intern at the time, so he was never home. When you're on call every other night, or even every third or fourth night, the issue is not quality time, the issue is absence. A fashionable view these days is that it is the first three months or the first six months or perhaps the first year that are crucial in a child's development, and that if this time is respected, then the parents can resume their normal activities without concern. Even if this is true, which I doubt, consider that a forty-hour week would be a half-time internship. Some medical couples, especially when both are in medicine, assert that if you can pay top dollar for child care it doesn't matter how much time the parents are away. Doctors in practice are indeed fortunate to make enough money to give their children the best, although not many house officers are so lucky. Usually the wife is stuck at home, pining all the more for her husband because she has an infant as a constant reminder of the value of adult companionship. Even if the family can afford live-in help, however, there comes a point where the children might as well be nanny's except for their privileged financial status.

I may sound old-fashioned, harping on child-care questions, but this is an issue that does not melt away, even after training. Traditionally, women doctors have chosen such fields as psychiatry or radiology where nine-to-five hours are the norm. Or they work part-time, which contributes to the great discrepancy between the mean salaries of men and women in medicine. The female medical entrepreneur is a rare bird, and I think will continue to be so, as long as children remain important. Fields that require long training, such as neurosurgery, are opening up to women, as is academic medicine to a certain extent, but the women I know who are serious about such careers have either had their children early or don't plan to. One physician on our faculty confided to me that she felt childbearing was an overrated experience. She is divorced and her husband has custody of the children.

Trends in medical practice are currently more amenable to women. Now, for the first time, there are slightly more salaried physicians than fee-for-service practitioners. In addition, with the predicted doctor glut of the 1980s and 1990s, half-time work will provide more slots for more bodies. In fact, I am cynical enough to believe that the larger presence of women in medical schools is tolerated partly because we are not perceived as the same manpower threat as an equal number of men. We may be moving closer to the Russian model—there, women make up the bulk of care-giving physicians—but the status of such practitioners is low compared to those in the university. The traditional town-gown rivalry in the United States has pitted the brilliance of the lab jocks against the money of the private practitioner. Now that the lab doctor has investments in genetic engineering and the physicians outside are tending to receive salaries for more circumscribed responsibility, the balance may shift.

The child you bear fourth year does not disappear when you enter internship, nor necessarily become less demanding. This is the time to establish your priorities toward family, whatever the family may be. Medicine is a greedy taskmaster. It will take as much of your soul as you are willing to give. So be honest as you assess your long hours in the hospital. Is that where you feel most alive? Or are you like my fellow resident, who vowed at the end of his training to never set foot in a hospital? There is room in medicine for both kinds of doctors, but if the I.C.U. monitors are playing your song, it is probably not a nursery rhyme.

Compared to some of our more adventurous classmates who forged ahead with their life's business—mating and procreating—during the clinical years, my husband and I stumbled along like lost children in the woods. We tried to keep a cat but abandoned the effort when we realized that, in any given twenty-four-hour period, neither of us could be relied upon to be home long enough to feed her. We argued over who could take time off to cash a check so that we could buy food and deferred the laundry as long as possible by purchasing two weeks' worth of underwear apiece. Our adjustment was particularly rough because we were both on call, usually on opposite schedules. If we were both in the hospital every third night, he would be away Monday, I Tuesday, both home Wednesday, although I might have been up all night. His turn again Thursday, mine Friday, etc. The only way we could have totally coordinated our schedules was to have taken every clerkship together, which I could not have tolerated. We did do the same clerkships at the same time at different hospitals, in order to have vacations together. Vacations were not always that much better because we planned them for when we thought we would be the most tired, after the rigorous clerkships, which meant we often didn't have time to make reservations or research points of interest. If we wanted to get away, rather than just sleep, we had to drive, to save money. It was not unusual for us to put several thousand miles on the car in one week.

I was insufferable without sleep and knew it, so I insisted on spending most of my free time trying to catch up. I didn't learn to live with fatigue until internship, and then only by accident. I noticed that my fellow interns, who were single, made dates for the nights after they had been on call, knowing full well that they might find themselves stepping out after thirty-six hours awake. I thought they were crazy at first: I never planned to do anything but crash. But I soon realized that while they may have been crazy, they were crazy happy, while I was depressed and obsessed with my fatigue. So we too started making plans, even if one of us had been up all night. Often we only lasted through dinner; movies were a waste of money because we just fell asleep. There can be a certain euphoria to sleep deprivation. My personal triumph of will occurred on my birthday during internship year. I had literally been on my feet for two days and one night, but when I dragged home at seven dreaming only of bedclothes, I found my husband and another couple waiting to take me out to a fancy Italian restaurant as a surprise. A year earlier I would have begged off, but hell, it was my birthday. I slapped some water on my face and partied.

Spouses should not get into the habit of counting on a live wire when their doctor comes home, however. All that waiting creates unreasonable expectations: It is not going to be all better when he gets home, because he's most likely to be grumpy and unresponsive. Sleep deprivation is like alcohol: If things have gone well, I can be very up, until the crash. But my judgment is impaired; I don't necessarily remember what I do or say and I can be quite paranoid. Driving home some nights, I was scarcely able to change lanes because I was sure all the car lights were coming at me.

As a spouse myself, I am sorry to report that waiting doesn't get any easier as the years roll by. One breakthrough for me in this regard was the realization that I did not always have to be at home when my husband arrived, even if I hadn't seen him for two days. Rather than cooking a meal he would merely inhale on the way to bed, sometimes I would go visiting, or run errands and let him fend for himself. It may sound cruel, but I think it was a relief for him to be able to crash without guilt every now and then. This strategy is more difficult with children, but equally valuable. My inclination is always to hand my husband the baby as he walks in the door, but realistically I know that one night on call equals two nights away. Remember this when choosing a clerkship or a house-staff program, for the difference between every fourth night call and every third night is greater than it first appears. Every fourth night call doubles one's free time, since there are two nights after the crash night, instead of one.

Anything that can divert the waiting spouse is a plus during the clinical years. Go to the movies with friends: If you don't have friends, go alone. I am always surprised at married women who tell me they wouldn't dream of going to a movie alone because they are still wedded to the high school mentality dictating that a girl without a date must nurse her unpopularity at home. There is a legitimate safety issue sometimes, but be sure you're not just making excuses. Schedule yourself for evening classes or work overtime sometimes, even if it occasionally cuts into your time together. All my male colleagues had hobbies that they continued to pursue rather than plan every free second with their wives, yet often their wives would not feel the same freedom to entertain themselves. It's bad enough putting one life on hold for the duration; no point in doubling the misery.

The most important advice is to try to maintain perspective. Every argument should include an analysis, "Is it us, or is it the situation?" When every second counts, each oversight is magnified. It wouldn't matter so much about forgetting to put out the garbage before work if someone were coming home soon enough to get it out before the house is condemned as a health hazard. A night out with the boys doesn't sound excessive unless that's half of the nights he's home that week. Couples who spent years working out an equitable distribution of household chores now have to renegotiate every trip to the laundromat, because suddenly one partner's routine is unpredictable. If you can concentrate on the big picture when the household details are driving you bananas, you will be able to hang on. Not that the hours will improve much in the foreseeable future (or ever), but having a little spare change to send the shirts to the laundry or to hire someone to clean the house or watch the baby makes all the difference in the world. An apartment with a dishwasher and washers and dryers in the building is worth a year of marriage counseling.

As for the student herself, let me start with the basics. We tell our patients that it is important to eat sensibly, rest and exercise regularly, yet we skip meals, stay up all night, and then say we're too tired to exercise. Partly, it is not our fault. But there is rarely a clinical crisis so grave that a student can't be spared. When I first started a medicine clerkship at the veterans' hospital, a cynical intern advised me, "Never miss a meal for a vet." Now, that's a fairly callous instruction, but it contains a kernel of truth. Early on, we revel in our self-importance and pretend we're indispensable when it just isn't so. It would probably serve the whole team better for you as a student to slip out to the cafeteria and grab some food for everyone. Of course, medical people learn to eat incredibly fast, so it's likely everyone could make it if they tried. The capacity to wolf down a meal while discussing someone's innards truly separates the men from the boys.

So eat, at the very least. Better yet, take your lunch sometimes. Avoiding hospital food allows you a measure of control over your life, and you can pack food with fiber and taste for less than you would spend on the cafeteria pabulum. If you are a food junkie like me (and an awful lot of other doctors, I've noticed), the texture of real whole-wheat bread, not that tan stuff, is enough to transport you out of the hospital momentarily. A chunk of Brie and a piece of a baguette satisfies the soul for about the same cost as a cheeseburger. When I was totally disgusted with my life, I would pack dinner, too; usually there's a refrigerator without urine specimens that you can use and often there is a microwave to warm an entrée. One of my friends used to pack lunch, dinner, and breakfast: I was never so ambitious, but I admired the spirit.

Exercise is tougher to fit in, but just as rewarding. I took up running because I could do it anytime, alone if necessary, and safely enough. I wouldn't run after dark, but many guys I know did: Some would be out at five A.M. training for marathons. I found it easiest to slip out in the middle of the day, at lunchtime or a little after. As house staff, we would hold each other's beepers for an hour, a practice that, while not condoned officially, was well known.

As a student you shouldn't have any responsibility problems, but you can't pretend you're studying for that hour.

In some families, anything that keeps the medical partner away, even another hour a day, becomes a point of contention. While my husband never objected, I only tried to run long distances once, when he temporarily took up running with me and we were trying for a marathon. We were both relieved when injuries stopped us about a month before the race: Frankly, a three-hour run is not my idea of how to spend Sunday morning. My male friends generally felt they "deserved" the time it took to train. I understood their point: After consorting with the weak and the maimed all day long, it is damned reassuring to stretch out, young and strong. But I have identified a third-year-resident syndrome that can crop up fourth year or any time that the anxiety and workload at the hospital decreases temporarily. Instead of devoting the found time to loved ones, we doctors have to drive ourselves to excel in another area of human endeavor. We're like windup toys that can't wind down. Watch out for it.

When overwhelmed by a patient suffering total body failure, I was taught to ask, "If I could fix one thing for you, what would it be?" That question would force all but the most diffuse patients to focus on a chief complaint, which would give the physician a fighting chance at unraveling their problem. If I could fix one thing for the clinical students, it would be their self-esteem. The pressure to conform to the myth of the tireless physician oblivious to life outside the hospital is quickly internalized, because no one wants to be, heaven forbid, a bad doctor. And if you eat, drink, and breathe the hospital, naturally the approval of those in charge seems all important. For some of us nontraditional types, however, that approval never comes. Or it comes at the expense of some deepset convictions, like those of my friend James.

Toward the end of third year, my husband informed me that it wasn't normal to come home every night and cry. So I went to a psychiatrist, who told me basically that medical school was tough, that it was tougher for women and blacks, and that I was coping pretty well. All the raw nerves were part of the program. Eventually I stopped crying. I allowed myself to laugh at the onerousness of the physician's role. As house officers we joked about spending "just another day in paradise" or described our work as "saving lives and stamping out disease." I came to terms with the fact that, given a choice, doctors and patients would always make eye contact with the male sitting next to me, because he "looked like a doctor." No matter that he might be the pharmacy student on the team. I realized that what I liked about medicine, helping people, was not necessarily the goal of the high-tech blitz that dominated the teaching center. And encounter after encounter convinced me finally that one reason that I had such difficulty modeling myself on my professors was that they might as well inhabit another planet, so distant were they from my realities.

One day at the beginning of my surgery clerkship, my preceptor called me in for a chat. He said he wanted to get to know me as a person, so he could write a more complete evaluation. I thought that was laudable, if weird. He asked me what my hobbies were, what I did with my free time. Always at a loss for impressive pastimes, I told him that I read quite a bit and had recently joined a women's group. I knew the latter was a mistake as soon as it was out of my mouth, but he passed over it, not bothering to write it down. He asked me what I read.

"Novels," I replied.

"What do you mean, novels?" I fell silent, stunned. "Do you mean you choose books from the best-seller list?"

"No. You know, novels." I was desperate. "Like you used to read in high school." He didn't write that down, either. Flailing around, I remembered that I had heard he was a runner. "I jog about ten miles a week." At least he wrote that down. "And I just tried cross-country skiing for the first time."

"Did you like skiing?"

"Oh, yes," I replied, relieved.

"Do you ski downhill?"

"No, I haven't tried that."

"Why not?"

"Well, it's rather expensive to start out downhill, if you've never done it before. All the equipment and the lift tickets . . ." I trailed off because he was looking blank again.

"I never thought of it in terms of money." He paused. "You know, downhill skiing is a high-risk sport."

"Yes."

"Do you know what a high-risk sport is?"

"Well, I suppose it is a sport where you run a high risk of injury."

"Correct." He was getting at something, but I had no idea what. "Did you know that people who participate in high-risk sports have a lower rate of cardiovascular mortality than the general population?"

"No, I didn't."

"Well," he continued, exasperated. "Do you participate in any high-risk sports?"

"No, I suppose not."

That finished him. He stared at me a little more and then delivered the coup de grâce. "You know this interview was supposed to help you."

Mercifully, I don't remember what I replied to that. I probably apologized for existing. To this day I cannot figure how I could have helped my evaluation except by total prevarication. The bad news is that, in medical school, conversations like this matter. The good news is that, in the long run, they don't matter at all.

7

FOURTH YEAR: EXPLORING THE FIELD

If third year is life in the fast lane, fourth year is a six-lane highway, full of choices. You can continue in the fast lane if you like, taking many demanding ward clerkships called subinternships, but you can also change lanes and set your cruise control to a more leisurely pace, taking clerkships such as dermatology or radiology, in which showing up each day is about the level of commitment required. Or you can pull off the road entirely, if your requirements are finished, and graduate early, assuming you have some other means of support than financial aid. Some students arrange clerkships abroad: in Europe for specialty training in areas such as cardiology or neurology, or in Third World countries for hands-on intensive primary care. Students from abroad like to do clinical clerkships in the United States, since our training is often more practical than theirs. Fourth year presents options that vanish again until the end of your postmedical training. Yet unlike the kid in the candy store who is oblivious to next year's dental bill, the fourth-year student must tackle internship applications. That task is as unsavory as any application process, additionally weighted by the simultaneous choice of medical specialty. Not to speak of the irony of competing for a position that holds no intrinsic interest. You could explain to interviewers why you wanted to go to medical school, but no one in his right mind actually wants to be an intern.

As usual, the choices you make this year pertain to the year ahead. Only the most unpopular clerkships are available at this point, since most of clerkship scheduling was second year and you undoubtably filled in your electives shortly thereafter. My previous advice, to choose electives that are not necessarily in your career field, still stands. If you were overly enthusiastic and filled your schedule with subinternships, now is the time to try to wriggle out of some of them. Most of the time, dropping those clerkships at the last minute is pretty difficult because the ward in question needs your body despite your lack of expertise. And, believe me, none of your fellow students will want to pick up an extra intensive care unit slot once the internship choices are out. Nevertheless, one enterprising woman in our class managed to drop a subinternship at one hospital to receive pay for the same work at another where an intern had quit mid-year. She ruffled quite a few feathers but had her way.

Once again, let me assure you that you will be "prepared" for internship without doing the whole year in advance. If I could have scrounged airfare to Nepal, I would have gone for as much of the year as possible. As it was, I graduated in March and spent a delightful few months taking Spanish at a community college and reading every novel I could get my hands on. My husband had to stay enrolled in order for us to receive the financial aid that came in his name. Family therapists speak of the identified patient in a dysfunctional family—well, my husband was the identified pauper. So he took the easiest clerkships he could and we escaped on long weekends. We did have time between his graduation and start of internship to take a long camping trip through the Pacific Northwest. I have always attributed the perfect weather we enjoyed in that normally soggy part of the country to God's forbearance in the face of our imminent bondage. No need to destroy us twice.

If, like me, you tend toward the easy burnout, a relaxing fourth year is the best insurance that you will finish your internship. Every year, in every program, several interns bite the dust. The selection committees try to guard against this by choosing tough students, but sometimes the very student who performed brilliantly in the intensive care unit, the coronary care unit, the cancer ward, and the emergency room, simply can't face it all again. I will admit, however, that it looks better on your transcript to have a few heavy-duty clerkships early on fourth year and to serve as an apprentice weaver the second semester. And, as I mentioned before, any clerkship taken at another medical school to impress their internship selection committee must be finished before that committee meets in November and December. January is simply too late.

The true business of fourth year is selecting an internship, or more precisely, arranging for the internship of your choice to select you. This occurs through an amazing computerized system, the National Intern and Resident Matching Program, casually referred to as the Match. The concept of the Match is quite simple: Students rank internships by order of preference, internships rank students the same way, the two lists are thrown into the black box known as the computer, and each program secures the best interns who want to come. For example, let's say my first choice is the pediatrics program in Fairyland; my second, Dreamworld. Suppose then that as a good but not stellar student, I am among Dreamworld's top ten choices for their ten places, but Fairyland ranks me twentieth and has only five prestigious places to fill. If by some fluke there are not five students among the first nineteen Fairyland chosen who want their program, I will end up with my first choice. Otherwise, I will go to Dreamworld. I cannot refuse to go in a fit of pique, because the paper I signed to enter the Match is legally binding: I agreed to go where they send me. Otherwise, the internship programs could not be sure their manpower needs would be met. It will already have occurred to the more astute among you that it is possible that neither Fairyland nor Dreamworld will be interested if I am a truly poor student, in which case I will end up with no internship. This dreaded eventuality is known as "not matching," happens infrequently, and will be discussed later.

The key to matching is to have a good sense of where you stand in your class and rank programs that are likely to rank you. At schools with grades, your class ranking may be obvious. Our school was on a pass-fail-honors system that obscured the rankings a bit, but it was clear that honors grades were necessary to apply to the top programs and I am firmly convinced that the dean had a numerical list as well. Membership in Alpha Omega Alpha, the medical school honor society comparable to the undergraduate Phi Beta Kappa, also gives your application a boost. Your entire academic career is summarized in the dean's letter that accompanies every application. And after all this information has been reviewed, the chiefs of the various services call their buddies across the country and say anything they were afraid to put in print. You also interview, but your school knows you better than you might think by now, and the interview is more for your information than theirs.

The match system was devised to prevent the chaotic scrambling for places that apparently used to occur every spring. Interviewers would "guarantee" a student a place, so the student would relax and then find himself with no internship. It is now specifically forbidden to promise places (or accept them) before the Match, but many of my friends swore they were offered places. In fact, it occurred so frequently that I wondered whether it was a matter of wishful hearing, especially since several friends were disappointed when the Match took place. At any rate, don't trust any offer made outside the Match, unless you have been exempted from the program.

The only common exemption is the one that applies to couples. Couples may, if they so choose and are able, make a deal outside the Match in order to end up in the same place. My husband and I went this route, so we knew where we would be several months before our classmates. Going outside the Match limited our options: Many programs would not consider us, although they encouraged us to apply through the Match. The problem seems to be that if there are only fifteen internship slots, most programs are not willing to gamble two of them on a couple from outside. We were offered positions only at our own medical school and one other in the state. We were counseled by some to leave our school for fear of becoming too parochial. If one or the other of us had been terrifically ambitious, we might have felt we were "settling" in some sense, rather than finding our true worth on the open market. As it was, we decided that two places in hand were worth all the possibilities in the bush. Had we been unable to sell ourselves outside the Match, we would have known early enough to cast our lot with the masses, which was a comforting thought as the "no-way" responses to our proposal rolled in.

It is also possible to match as a couple, although it is a somewhat distasteful process. The first step is that one person must be identified to the computer as the "more important" partner, that is, the one who will be matched independently. Then the computer matches the "less important" partner to the mate. In order to maximize the chances of ending up together, it makes sense to designate the weaker candidate the more important partner. For instance, if the weaker student is accepted at any one of the institutions on the couple's rank list, they will match together, assuming that programs ranking the poorer student would automatically rank the better one also. If, on the other hand, the stronger student is the independent agent, he could conceivably match only to programs that did not rank his partner. But the whole idea of designating a more and less important partner made my stomach turn, especially since I was the partner with the weaker grades.

When we were wrestling with these painful prospects, I was advised by several people to consider matching in a separate field, such as pediatrics, which was, after all, more suitable for a woman. I liked pediatrics, but I hadn't done particularly well in it: The fact that I even entertained the possibility of a career in the field is a measure of my panic that we might not end up together. I put aside such thoughts when I realized that if my husband dropped dead at the end of our residency, I would be a pediatrician, alone. I am not sure now that it would have been easier in two fields than in one, anyway. Fortunately, we were both good students, so that neither one of us had to do much sacrificing. I shudder to think what might have ensued had our records been vastly different.

Those who don't match are so informed the day before everyone else learns of their fate, so they can scramble for any leftover places. In the good old days, there were more slots than interns to fill them, but not today. Yet it seems that certain reasonable programs may not fill, so failure to match is not the end of the world. It is definitely not cool, however, so if you manage to find a place within twenty-four hours, I would say there is no need to give the gory details to the public. Your best friends will realize that Cook County in Chicago was not at the top of your list, but just explain airily to the rest of the world that you wanted the true county hospital experience or that you suspect you're a Midwesterner in your soul.

Those are the mechanics of the Match. The problem is that, in order to rank a list of programs, the student has to decide what field he or she wants to enter, where he or she wants to live for the training period, and perhaps where he or she wants to practice, since it is easier to establish contacts for practice opportunities locally. If the training program to which you match has a national reputation in your field or if you plan to change programs after internship, it may not matter where you start. Certain programs, such as anesthesia, radiology, dermatology, and ophthalmology, accept students to residency programs outside of the Match, only stipulating that the student complete some sort of internship first. So a budding pediatric radiologist would apply to radiology programs third or fourth year and enter into the Match for a pediatric internship. Students who set their sights on internal medicine, surgery, psychiatry, obstetrics, or pediatrics generally match for an internship-residency package in order to avoid a second selection process. Some programs, especially general surgery, it seems, have a pyramid system, with more places at the internship level than at the third- or fourth-year resident level. The expectation is that a few residents will want to leave the field either for subspecialty training (orthopedics, ear, nose, and throat) or another kind of medicine. If that doesn't happen or if you don't cut the mustard, you may be dropped and have to scramble again.

In the old days, when there was less undergraduate clinical work, it was common to choose a rotating internship, which would allow some exposure to all the major fields. Such a system allowed a more rational residency choice and made for a well-rounded clinician. While there are still some rotating internships available, the general practitioner who hangs out his shingle after his internship is a vanishing species. Legally, it's still possible, since a license to practice is granted after satisfactory completion of an internship and certification by the National Board or the FLEX exam. Of course, you can take a rotating internship with plans to continue in a residency, but then you have to be sure that your internship will include enough months of your chosen specialty to allow you to be board certified in that field.

Another theoretical option for the terminally undecided is to apply to two kinds of residencies at once and let the Match decide whether you end up an obstetrician or a general surgeon. Don't do it. Even if you absolutely must end up in one particular city, apply to all the programs in one field rather than the best ones in two. The reason is that if the programs get wind of it, both of them will be inclined to rank the student who knows his own mind higher, so you might end up shut out with good credentials. Given departmental barriers, it might appear that it would be easy to keep one set of programs ignorant of your other applications but gossip gets around.

The decision to reject all those options that made medicine such an appealing career choice can be agonizing. Just remember that, at best, clerkships are merely a window onto a specialty. The view may be quite limited, even distorted. In order to provide perspective, try to imagine where you would like to be and what you would like to be doing in ten years. Then seek out a few doctors who seem to be living your fantasy. Within academia, the only role models are academics. If you envision yourself as a general surgeon in a small community, you may have to contact an alumnus or a friend of a sympathetic professor. But make the effort, to avoid surprise later. There's a lot to medicine besides intellectual challenge: politics, government, grants, hospital privileges, business management.

Another creative way to approach a specialty is to imagine how you would feel about treating that field's problem patient. Orthopedics may be all fun in the hospital, patching up athletes and inserting artificial joints, but bread-and-butter orthopedics includes treating chronic lower back pain, a discouraging ailment if there ever was one, and more than a fair share of litigious patients out for disability or compensation from accidents. Oncology is an exciting field when you can offer new therapy to patients with leukemia or lymphoma, but the most common cancer among men is lung, which is still a death sentence, and among women is breast, an emotional landmine. Kids are fun and generally healthy, but there is no human being more distraught than the parent of a sick child, nor anyone more likely to call the doctor in the middle of the night "just to be sure."

Finally, compare your temperament to those of the residents you have met: Ask them why they chose their field. If you don't get along with the elderly, internal medicine is not for you. If you can't get up in the morning, forget anesthesia. If you are a cook who serves scampi as an appetizer, chateaubriand and asparagus for an entrée, and chocolate mousse for dessert, you should be a surgeon: As such you will be much appreciated for sophisticated, largely standardized procedures. Sure, you can botch an operation, just as you can burn the chateaubriand, but in both cases success is largely dependent on selection and execution with a reasonable amount of care. If you prefer to experiment with ethnic dishes even with guests coming and don't care that they are not necessarily bowled over by your presentation, you can risk primary care, where the patients are a grab bag and the rewards less generous.

Other thoughts. Obstetrics and gynecology is a field that gracefully combines surgery and primary care: The only problem is that you have to turn your back on half the human race. If you are a woman, definitely consider obstetrics and gynecology. The male gynecologists are positively courting their female colleagues these days because so many women choose a practice for the woman partner. Perhaps grateful patients keep you happy: Then consider ophthalmology or oncology. If you can restore a patient's eyesight, he will sing your praises unto the hills. And if you stand by a cancer patient after he has been rejected by family, friends, and often his own doctor, he will swear you are the greatest physician on earth, regardless of your success or lack thereof in treating his disease. If you are a city gal interested in old-fashioned family practice, you may find yourself facing a move to the country, for in some urban areas family practitioners can't obtain hospital privileges to deliver babies or assist in surgery because the specialists have a monopoly on the market. Urban patients, too, are used to seeing a gynecologist for a pelvic, an ear, nose, and throat doctor for ear wax, and an orthopedic surgeon for tennis elbow. People give lip service to the wonders of a general doctor who can treat the whole body when they are well, but when they fall ill, they want the best specialist in the business.

Finally, don't forget pathology. It's not as exciting as it is portrayed on television, but it must be intellectually satisfying to actually know the answer. As they say, internists know all but do nothing, surgeons know nothing and do all, pathologists know all and do all, but it's too late. The advantage of pathology is that it is a lucrative nine-to-five field involved with clinical medicine but shielded from the demands of John Q. Public. As an intern, I used to hide in the bone-marrow room, a little cubbyhole off the main lab where the pathologists reviewed the bone-marrow slides. Whenever I was involved with a patient who had a bone-marrow study or did one myself, I would slip down to study the slides with a pathology resident who was always tolerant of my ignorance: I suspect the pathologists welcomed the chance to chat. All was serene, and I felt I could linger there legitimately since I was learning about my patient. Anyway, you can only spend so much time in the bathroom.

It is probably wisest to address questions of prestige head-on when choosing a training program and a field for your life's work. At the house-staff level, academic training programs—those connected with a medical school—are more prestigious than those in private hospitals. If you are planning to go into academic medicine, you should not even consider a nonacademic program. If you want to be a clinician, the choice is yours, as long as your grades are solid.

The university setting offers intellectual stimulation from professors who teach you and students whom you are required to teach. Your fellow house staff, who are probably the single most important influence in your training, are likely to be sharper, although their first love may not be clinical medicine. In a private program, you generally manage your patients with private doctors, who of course are not preselected the way a faculty is. On the other hand, you will enter the real world at the start of your internship rather than at the conclusion of your training, so you will have opportunities to shine for potential partners and, very importantly, to measure yourself against the standard of the community. Academically trained physicians tend to be chronically insecure, after having all the "experts" look over their shoulders. Although they are more rigorously trained, they are less confident of their abilities. It is easier to land a fellowship in a university if you trained in one, so you need to think ahead. One student may decide that his priority is to live in a particular city and apply to academic and nonacademic programs there, hoping for the former but willing to settle for the latter. Another may feel temperamentally unsuited to the private hospital because tact is not his strong suit. A third may prefer the more relaxed pace of most private hospitals. If you are a good student, you will be encouraged to stay in the university, but try to make up your own mind. I stayed at the university and was happy, but I remained a small fish in a big pond, unlike some of my friends who left.

You might as well also consider the prestige of the medical specialties you are contemplating, because you will have to live with your decision later. Don't kid yourself that prestige and money don't matter as you're choosing a specialty. Fortunately, many doctors feel that other aspects of their profession matter more, but it's no accident our society is top-heavy with surgeons and subspecialists. To start at the top, surgeons are held in high regard and well paid. Within surgery, the "cleaner" specialties, such as cardiac and neurosurgery, outrank the plumbers (urologists) and proctologists. Internists are better respected by other doctors than by patients, who don't understand what we do. They don't forget the guy who "cut on them," but they rarely remember who made the diagnosis. Medical subspecialists outearn general internists several times over because they can perform such procedures as endoscopies, bronchoscopies, and cardiac catheterizations. Surgeons may not be closer to God, but anyone who breaches the integument is closer to the insurance carriers.

Psychiatrists, by contrast, are better respected by patients than other doctors, who tend to treat them as glorified social workers. I have heard gynecologists dismissed as butchers by surgeons and as birdbrains by internists, but I am convinced their reputation suffers for dealing exclusively with women. Some doctors even argue that the field should be abolished because women will receive second-class care as long as they are segregated as patients. That makes some theoretical sense to me, but such a move would require a radical restructuring of medical education; male internists and surgeons are not ready for us. Pediatricians and family practitioners have a real image problem, reflected in their low level of remuneration. The jury is still out on the attempt to upgrade the general practitioner into a family specialist but it is not a field to choose if you seek the adulation of your peers. The physicians who specialize in order to master a field often have no appreciation of the effectiveness of a good generalist. Other doctors tend to view radiology, pathology, dermatology, and anesthesiology as cushy; these specialties are low profile with the public, which sometimes fails to perceive their practitioners as real doctors. Not to belabor the point, every field has its public and professional image, which may or may not mesh with yours. Look into it.

Do consider the sort of environment you will be working in as an intern, just as you did when choosing where to take your clerkships. As a student, I remember meeting a pleasant woman during the first days of her internship and being shocked to learn that she quit after a month. (I was shocked just to learn you could quit!) Rumor had it that all her training had been in Utah, where the largely Mormon population eschews drugs and liquor. When she realized how much of her time would be spent temporarily sobering up self-destructive weirdos, she just split.

The environment for your family is important, too. I once asked a resident's Southern-born wife if she and her toddler daughter liked San Francisco: She replied by telling me about the gay prostitute on her block who solicited business by masturbating in the window. She wasn't going to settle in the Bay Area, no matter what. A more common problem is that the job market is such that a short move may be hard or impossible for the working spouse. Peripatetic academicians can approach military men in moves advancing their careers: They need partners who are either self-sufficient or selfless or both. At conferences, I am always struck by the fact that no matter where the speaker hails from, the medical slang is the same. Since the slang is not communicated in journals, it must reflect the movement of bodies.

So much for choosing an internship. Medical students don't handle uncertainty very well, so everyone is in a fair tizzy by Match day. The only way to describe the scene as the envelopes are opened is in romantic burlesque. Oh, what cries and tears of joy! What embracing and running back and forth from friend to friend asking where, and oh, heart! Repeating endlessly the happy news of a place well landed or bemoaning the cruel turn that had denied the soul's longing. Finally, after much consoling, confiding, and congratulations, the various parties of intimates retire to their favorite taverns, there to drown the previous trembling in the sweet relief of knowledge. But not before the quick telephone call to loved ones waiting, for they, too, had a stake in the day's unveiling.

Aside from internship applications, senior year offers an opportunity to direct your own education, something you may well have forgotten how to do over the last three years. First you have to practice saying, "I want," then tack on some infinitives. "I want to be able to read a cardiogram," says the internist. "I want to perfect my one-handed knot," adds the surgeon. "I want to master the developmental stages of infancy," chimes in the pediatrician. "I want to feel more confident about my pelvic exam," the gynecologist decides. Once you get started, setting your own educational goals is positively exhilarating.

Two of the most useful skills to work on fourth year are reading electrocardiograms and chest X rays. Gynecologists can get by without ever encountering these tests, I suppose, but most other clinicians need to make their acquaintance. Certainly, surgeons are not going to be offering authoritative electrocardiogram interpretations, but they need to know enough about them to recognize trouble, just as I need to know enough about abdominal pain to call for help. If after fourth-year cardiology and radiology clerkships you know how to approach the problem systematically and have effectively suppressed the urge to freak out when someone hands you an electrocardiogram tracing, you have done well.

Subinternships are a special category of clerkships that are closer to internships, as the name implies, than to the clinical work of the third year. A good fourth-year clinical clerk functions as an intern without pay, although he may be protected somewhat from the worst of the intern's lot. As a resident, I tried to apportion patients so the student was not totally overwhelmed or saddled with drunk after drunk. Nevertheless, the subinternship is the time to develop habits that will propel you through house-staff training. Now you must learn to be totally compulsive, if you are not already. Buy yourself a clipboard and start making lists of what you have to do. As a long-time reader of what my husband derogatorily refers to as "home economics magazines," I recognized the technique as that recommended for efficient grocery shopping. To navigate quickly through a supermarket, you should arrange the list in categories: dairy, produce, meat, frozen foods. To navigate through a hospital, you need categories such as lab, X ray, i.v.s, dressings. It is more efficient to visit the X-ray department once and check four patients' films than to run back every hour for each one. Similarly, if there are three i.v.s to start, you might as well gather all that equipment once. The process of list making is nearly as important as the list itself; it is calming to be able to order catastrophe, if only on paper.

Keep an index card on each patient, stamped with each

one's addressograph, so you'll always know his or her hospital number. On it list age, admission date, problem list, and for a complicated patient, the dates of important hospital procedures. As an intern you will find yourself assuming the care of patients in their fourth or fifth hospital *month*. There's no way on earth you can remember what happened to the patient before you met him without a reminder, and like as not, no one will be able to locate the part of the chart that's been thinned after you review it when you come on service (if then). Also write down allergies. More than once, I have decided to give a patient a medicine to which he is allergic. There are safeguards against the medicine reaching the patient—the nurse and the pharmacist are supposed to check also—but the responsibility rests with the physician who writes the order.

As for orders, it is crucial that you learn to write clear, compassionate ones. Fourth-year students typically write the orders on their own patients, countersigned by an intern or resident. *Orders* is such an old-fashioned, autocratic term, but it is accurate. Your instructions as a doctor define the patients' lives and must be obeyed or else by hospital staff. Your patient quite literally cannot go to the bathroom without your say-so. When I first encountered this concept, I could not believe it. I thought, how dreadful for the patient, to so surrender his autonomy. It is also dreadful for the physician who must serve as a dictator in a police state. Mrs. Stewart has to follow a low-salt diet, Mr. Jones must be restrained, Mrs. Pratt can walk (or "ambulate," in hospital talk) only with assistance. No food for Mr. Lee until after his blood test, an enema for Mrs. Colvo before her sigmoidoscopy. Stick that one, turn this one, let that one go home. No wonder patients speak of being released, rather than discharged.

The formidable custodial role of the hospital requires orders for the protection of the gravely ill, but they drive anyone who isn't totally bananas. The trick in allowing patients a measure of self-respect is to anticipate their improvement. Write that it's okay for the cardiac patient to shower as soon as it is, not after he's been remanded to bed by the nurses following your bedrest order. Explain what preparation is involved before tests or surgery to avoid screams of "You're going to shave me *where*?" Allow the patient the most liberal diet possible. Hospital food is lousy and a two-gram sodium diet, which is often ordered routinely on anyone with a vaguely cardiac diagnosis, is abominable. My theory is that doctors encourage noncompliance at home with overzealous restriction in the hospital. Similarly, there is no reason to forbid a patient with lung cancer to smoke, as long as he's not on oxygen: The horse is out of the barn.

Also think of the nurses who have to carry out your orders. A nurse with ten patients can waste a lot of time measuring daily weights and urine output from patients who don't need to be followed so closely. Be quick to change orders as the patient stabilizes, or transfer patients to more intensive care if need be. Review the medication orders frequently and stop those prescriptions that are no longer needed.

Don't be afraid to be a little creative. The patient who complains of back pain doesn't necessarily need narcotics: Suggest that he get out of bed every so often and write for a heating pad. Hospital mattresses are uncomfortable. And every man who is able to stand deserves the chance, before you catheterize him for failure to urinate: Some guys just can't do it lying down. Modify your dosages of everything downward in the elderly. You can knock out an octogenarian for thirty-six hours with a dose of Valium that wouldn't even take the edge off a final exam for a college student. Be generous with pain medication where it is needed, however.

All this carping about orders may sound like much ado about nothing. It's true you'll never be graded on your orders. But staff and patients judge you by them and will respond in a spirit of cooperation to reasonable requests, while they will subvert unreasonable demands. Remember that the people who carry out your orders are almost as overworked as you are. I think another advantage of county hospital training is the downward mobility. In order to expedite matters, doctors perform the duties of patient escort, nurse, orderly, and technician. I wouldn't make a career of it, but it teaches humility.

Another item that many house officers consider indispensable is a little black book of personal notes. I kept one, filled with drug dosages and lists of differential diagnoses for common crises. I always carried a crib sheet for cardiac arrests, also, in case my mind went blank (never happened). I started compiling my notebook fourth year and kept it going until I was a senior resident. So I would recommend it for people like me who need the security of the written word. My husband, who is not a natural notetaker, panicked at the start of internship and bought a set of notes for house officers. I don't think he ever used them and they cost plenty.

How much of a library you carry with you depends, again, on your level of anxiety and how easily you can afford to replace the books when (not *if* but *when*) they are stolen. I carried only one, the *Manual of Medical Therapeutics*. As a student, I carried my ophthalmoscope with me until it was stolen, then I tried to get by as much as possible by borrowing from others. I did buy another one along the way, but I hated to bring it. Apparently, there is a vast market for hot medical equipment, so addicts put their hours in the hospital to good use. Every now and then the equipment is recovered: A friend once found his ophthalmoscope while checking the belongings of a John Doe who had arrived comatose. The gentleman had overdosed before he was able to sell it.

Fourth year is a good time to try to perfect your technique for a few simple procedures, even if you are not yet a master at performing them. Surgeons know that the right equipment, properly laid out, is critical to the successful operation. An internist tends to assemble equipment haphazardly and handicap himself with what is easily available rather than the ideal tool. The surgeon will yell bloody murder until he gets what he wants, wasting time that he then saves by doing it right the first time. Model yourself after the most meticulous resident you can find, then try to stick to his technique. Each new resident will try to teach you a better way, but no technique works without practice, and if you are constantly shifting gears, you'll never go forward.

Third year, I suggested you confine yourself to the textbook for reading. This year it is a good idea to wade a little into the stream of medical literature, while staying close to the safe shore of the now-familiar text. Start to collect classic review articles in your chosen field, but continue to ignore the kind of article that describes ten rats fed a yeast diet in New Guinea. If that turns out to be important, you'll hear it again, and chances are, it won't. If you have not yet subscribed to the major journal in your field, now is the time to do so. Resolve to save only the articles you want by tearing them out of the magazine and filing them: A stack of journals in the closet is useless. You can even start to play the academic game of roundsman-ship, quoting journals to support your point. It is the medical version of the game of Trivia, intended to show off how much you read more than to contribute to patient care. You can't avoid it entirely in any field, but surgeons justly accuse internists of mental masturbation, while internists consider neurologists and dermatologists the worst offenders. In general, the physicians who can offer the fewest therapeutic options read the most. Just remember, nobody loves a smart ass, so if your resident tells you to do something, don't quote back to him unless you're ready for an argument that may affect your grade.

As a subintern, you may feel you're beginning to know enough to help plan your patient's care or to disagree with your resident's suggestions. Here is an area in which you must carefully choose your battles because in almost all cases you will have to defer to your resident's greater experience. Medically my residents seemed infallible, but from time to time I had some serious ethical reservations about a course of treatment. Since everyone rotates, you may find yourself in the position of undoing with a second resident what you did with the first. When I rotated into the coronary care unit as a junior resident, I followed perhaps the most aggressive doctor in our group. He had been supervising a subintern caring for a ninety-year-old man who had suffered a massive heart attack. The man had total body failure: He was on a breathing machine, taking medicines to keep his blood pressure up, and on a dialysis machine because his kidneys had failed when he went into shock. I surveyed this scene with horror. Statistically, if this man had been forty years old, his chances of surviving to leave the hospital were about 20 percent. At ninety, with no living relatives and the best possible prospect an extended stay in a nursing home, I felt such vigorous intervention was completely unreasonable. I applied the "If this were my father would I . . . ?" rule and the answer was "No, no, no!"

But here was a fourth-year student, full of beans, eager to show me how well he could spout the numbers from all the machines. I tried to break it to him gently, to let him participate in the decision to back off, but I knew I was not going to continue on the course the other resident had set even if the student strenuously objected. We decided to stop dialysis, which meant the patient would die in a few days, barring a miracle. At that point, the former resident, a friend, barged in and screamed that if I was not willing to care for this patient, he would transfer him to his new service. The student and the nurses were taken aback and I was aghast at the scene we were creating, but I felt I was right just as strongly as he did. For once, I didn't have to worry about the accusation of laziness, which is always the interventionist's trump card: The patient would have been no trouble to keep alive because he was already on every machine possible. I stood my ground and let him die. What did the student really feel about the situation? It must have been very tough to let someone go whom he had worked so hard to save. Such cases are judgme. calls, questions of style, subject to interpretation. As a student, you have to try to appreciate various approaches until you can blaze your own trail.

The second part of the National Board falls fourth year: Take the test as close to your core (required) clerkships as possible, since your electives will probably not boost your performance. I remember it as sexist, full of hypochondriacal female patients, but easier than Part I. I studied nowhere near as much and did slightly better, probably because the problems were now patients.

Graduation marks the end of the first part of your medical training, the end of an era. My strongest emotion was astonishment that I had made it, that I was actually an M.D. Competitive to the end, I was somewhat envious of my husband's greater honors, but I clutched my degree like a talisman: No one could take that away from me. Though they tried. At a dinner to honor three distinguished graduates, one my husband, we were presented with name tags to wear for the evening. His read "Dr. So-and-So," mine read "Mrs. Him." I have never used his name, so that was a minor error, but I was damned if they were going to deny me my M.D. In order to avoid too much of a scene, I suggested we change the tag to "Dr." by merely crossing out the "Mrs." (There was no question of confusion because our first names were on the tags.) My gallant husband insisted that they make out a new tag with my own name and proper title. As we left the entryway, the wife of one of the department chairs berated me for asking for the change. "This is his night tonight, and you are his wife." If I had had any presence of mind, I would have suggested that "Dr." therefore be deleted from all the name tags except those of the honorees, or would have inquired whether my husband's name tag would have read "Mr." if I had won the prize. Instead, I slunk away. Later the main speaker made a jocular reference to the feminist presence, also aimed at me. Well, hell. I had played their game and finished, maybe not with highest honors, but with distinction. And I deserved credit that night, too, like every other physician in the room with "Dr." before his name.

As you start your house-staff training, you have an opportunity to be the physician of your dreams: sensitive to patients and co-workers, erudite, graceful under pressure, philosophical, humble. You can reject all the posturing and pomposity. That is, if you still care, doctor.

8
INTERNSHIP

On my first day as an intern, I received a name tag identifying me as a Resident I. Interns in other departments showed up with tags that read PG I, for postgraduate. Why the change in nomenclature? I'm still not sure. But whatever the name tag reads these days, the doctor in his first year of training after medical school is just a " 'tern," the buck private. The real residents are the guys who order you around, who jawbone about the patient's problems while you stand revising your scut list. The intern is always on the move, always in a hurry. He's the first one on the team in the hospital to pre-round and the last one to leave at night after signout. He sleeps the least and skips the most lectures. He's the bloodiest, from his spattered shoes to his stained white jacket. He carries the most paraphernalia: reflex hammers, tourniquets, syringes, i.v. tubing, gauze pads. And he's the most cynical. His overriding goal is to discharge patients, through the door if possible or through the morgue if not. "Treat 'em and street 'em," because there're always more on the way.

"Take a deep breath at the beginning of the year and hold it until it's over," a friendly resident advised me as I started. So I cut off most of my hair, donned my whites, and abandoned any previous attempts to lead a normal life. When I was in the hospital, I didn't think about leaving. I pretended that there was no outside world, because trying to work harder to leave earlier inevitably led to frustration when a crisis delayed departure once again. I forgot birthdays, I missed movies, I heard news days after it occurred, as though I had been backpacking in the mountains. I lost a year of life in the United States when I lived abroad; I lost another one as an intern.

Looking around me, I could tell others dealt with the experience differently. Those who had families outside of medicine could not totally ignore them. Perhaps there were interns who went food shopping for the week or checked out library books. Not me. I decided that for once in my life I was not going to be handicapped by running the household. I wanted to go for it, just like a man. I did not think I was capable of being both an intern and a person, and I had to be an intern. I think this attitude kept me from going crazy, because it eliminated all potential conflict. I expected no free time, so an afternoon off was a bonus. I did not try to see my husband, so if we both happened to be home it was a party. My friends were fellow interns, so I never lacked for company. Getting the job done was all that mattered.

By creating my own *Brigadoon* at the university hospital, I was open to all the seduction of internal medicine. Since I only did one internship, I can't speak for my method in other fields. My night call averaged every third night, which was similar to the schedule in pediatrics and obstetrics at our hospital. The surgeons took call every other night and you could hear them boasting in the halls, "The only trouble with being on call every other night is that you miss half the cases." It took every fiber of my will and dense blinders for me to make it through my internship. I can't conceive of the effort theirs required. Human beings are adaptable creatures to survive not nature but their own absurd constructs.

As a university hospital intern, I spent nine of my twelve months on services there, but I started in the emergency room at the county hospital. It was an odd beginning, because only two university medical interns rotated there at a time, so I missed the initial bonding of the group. In the emergency room, interns from medicine, surgery, and family practice rotated interchangeably. It was my last opportunity to sew lacerations and observe trauma management; it was the surgeon's last opportunity to watch the treatment of medical emergencies. The trauma exposure repelled me, and I did not compete with the other interns to stick and cut those patients. I tried to follow how the chief assessed the injuries and I jumped whenever he barked at me, but my heart wasn't in it. I preferred to find a semicomatose drunk with a nice long head laceration and secrete myself in a side pocket, shaving, cleaning, and sewing the wee hours away. To my surprise, children were great minor trauma patients. While their parents wrung their hands, ten-year-olds would supervise my work, begging for as many stitches as possible so that they could brag about them at school. Less pleasant were the intravenous drug abusers with skin abscesses from dirty needles. Opening those abscesses hurt, even with local anesthesia, and no one has less pain tolerance than a narcotics addict. Or a greater supply of foul epithets. There was precious little teaching when the emergency room was busy, but there was lots of practice. I miss minor procedures now as an internist; nothing I do professionally requires the mind-emptying concentration of sewing.

On the medical side of the emergency room, the excitement came from the patients who were dead on arrival, with no visible sign of trauma, from heart attack, respiratory arrest, stroke, suicide, drowning, smoke inhalation, drug overdose. We tried to raise the dead for twelve hours a day, in between treating everything from abdominal pain to sore throats to threatened abortions. Most of the month, like most of the year, is a blur now, but I do remember recognizing pulmonary edema by myself for the first time. The resident was busy with another intern at a resuscitation, and I was left to mind the motley assortment of patients under medical evaluation. The nurses wheeled in a patient who was sitting bolt upright on the guerney, pale, blue, sweating and swollen, breathing forty times a minute. It is conventional to describe whether a patient is in mild, moderate, or severe distress; here was my first real live severe. He couldn't wait for the resident. Automatically, I began to look for a vein to start an i.v., and as the nurse finished writing his vital signs on the guerney sheet, the right drugs came to me: furosemide, morphine, oxygen. It was a great relief to me to learn that studying worked, that I would be able to recognize diseases I had never seen before if I knew their descriptions well enough. Medical school hadn't convinced me. After a brief exam that confirmed my initial impression, I started therapy that the resident okayed on his return.

The emergency room of a big city hospital is like no

other place on earth. We used to call the waiting room for the veterans' hospital clinics purgatory, because there the patients waited for their fate to be decided. Admission to heaven or back to the hell of the real world. The county hospital, too, provides a haven for a large population of derelicts who know that if they can just act sick enough to be admitted they can count on three squares and clean sheets. Some days it seems that the whole world is high on one substance or another. Prostitutes roll in next to dowagers who keeled over at luncheon. Every day brings a new instant quadriplegic from a motorcycle accident, usually a teen-ager. And a couple of "found on floors" or "in garbage can" people, last seen forty-eight hours before, now covered with excrement and vermin, clinging to life. At midnight supper, we could compare "you won't believe what I saw" stories over the remains of dinner. What a scene that was, from eleven-thirty to one, maybe fifty house staff, no one over forty, clustered near the kitchen in the enormous cafeteria now dark around the perimeter. Our whites reflected the overhead fluorescent rays in an eerie island of cold light. The services sat together, table-hopping for consults, plotting strategy for the rest of the night. We lingered as long as we dared, or as the beepers and sirens allowed, loud-mouthing to keep the streaming misery downstairs at bay.

My next three rotations, to the metabolic ward, the cancer ward, and the private service kept me from the meat of the internship, the staff service, but turned out to be the most difficult for me in the end. Not the metabolic ward, where patients with exotic diseases of hormone excess or deficiency were scheduled for admissions that ran largely on protocols. That was a respite from the emergency room— "from the ridiculous to the ridiculous," I described it to those who asked. We averaged two or three admissions a *week*. Most of the time, the ward team, swollen with students, outnumbered the patients. The highlights of the rotation were the weekly chats with one of the senior researchers. Everyone dreaded them, because he actually asked us to think as research biologists, to try to re-create experimental avenues that would explore clinical problems. I dreaded those talks as much as anyone, afraid I would look stupid, yet I treasured the experience of directed speculation, one I had not had since undergraduate days. I also enjoyed the setting. He would crowd us, seated, into his book-lined office, and a cafeteria employee, whom he thanked by name each session, would bring in coffee. He served us ceremoniously in china cups. We all drank coffee like water at conferences but it was always self-serve, in Styrofoam. I think it was a measure of our discomfiture that every week someone managed to spill coffee all over, if not break the cup. Unfailingly gracious, the investigator would mop up and continue his Socratic discourse. We strained to follow him, perspiring from the coffee and the stuffy room, as tongue-tied as beginning language students. The analogy is apt, for we were beginners in scientific reasoning after years of Pavlovian memorization. I smile even now to think of that physician attempting in his courtly manner to reveal the beauty of scientific inquiry to us philistines.

The private service and the cancer service had one thing in common: Call was every fourth night, all by myself. A third-year medical resident was available in the hospital for consultations if necessary, but I knew I would lose face by calling too much. Night admissions were supposed to be rare on both services, but I managed to receive more than my share. In addition, the patients I was covering, that is, babysitting for the other physicians on the service, were complicated and demanding. On the private service, I was continuously exasperated as well as overwhelmed. One twenty-two-year-old prima donna had her husband call a pediatric anesthesiologist when the nurse couldn't start an i.v. in her arm rather than call me, the covering M.D. Imagine how happy I was to try to explain to the anesthesiologist, greatly annoyed at being disturbed, why this woman with perfectly accessible, normal-size veins felt she required his services. I apologized and started the line. Another time a patient refused to accept her private duty nurse because she was black. I am light enough so that she did not realize that the doctor she was complaining to was also black. The worst of it, though, was always being caught in the crossfire between the patient and the private physician. The patient would claim that Dr. So-and-so had promised her that the hospital kitchen would dress her salad only with walnut oil; Dr. So-and-so when finally reached on his yacht would deny it; and both of them would speak to me as though I were addled.

On the cancer service, the patients were too desperately ill to play such games, but on the nights alone I faced crisis after crisis. My first night on call, a young woman with terminal breast cancer suddenly developed more difficulty breathing. The metastasized tumor had collapsed her lung before, so eventually we had discussed how to manage this on rounds. I was not to call the surgeons to place a chest tube, the standard procedure, because the tube is painful and she was not expected to live out the week. I was just to stick a needle into her chest myself, let out the free air, and hope that the lung would reexpand. Well, I had drawn fluid off the pleural space several times as a student, but I had never attempted this maneuver, so I chickened out and called the third-year resident to make sure he agreed. I could tell he was a little skeptical, but we went ahead and did it, releasing the trapped air in the chest. Unfortunately, the patient developed a relatively common complication of air under the skin, but since there was no suction to help draw off the air as a chest tube would have provided, the air traveled under the skin of her face, arms, and chest until she looked like a balloon and sounded like puffed-rice cereal when her upper body was touched.

Most nights, I had to administer chemotherapy under protocols I read like a cookbook, except with less comprehension. We gave the chemotherapy at night so that the patients would sleep through some of their nausea. At that time, we had to mix all the drug solutions, which might involve drawing out the drug from ten small vials into a syringe then diluting it with saline. Some of the drugs were caustic, like the red liquid we called the Red Death, so I was extra careful. The dosages all had to be calculated in milligrams per kilogram, and I might have three patients receiving therapy in addition to the twenty I was covering. One night I was running chemotherapy on the fourteenth floor, the twelfth floor, and the eleventh floor, barely finishing mixing and administering one dose before I had to run to the next. The guy on fourteen had endured such disfiguring surgery for head and neck carcinoma that he didn't want his children to see him anymore, he confided tearfully as I hung the intravenous bottle and checked the line. The cancer was not under control, so his oncologist felt he should try the chemotherapy. He committed suicide later during that admission, and I remember actually wishing he had done it before my night on call.

As bad as the nights were, the days offered no respite.

We called one room the T.M. Room, for Thorazine and morphine, the drugs we were pushing to try to alleviate some of the pain of the women inside. One of them was a Cuban with the most beautiful blue eyes I have ever seen. I see them still in nightmares, full of pain, asking us over and over again why God did not want her. Another patient, just my age, dying of an obscure kidney tumor, would beg me not to give her chemotherapy because moving her arm enough for me to set the tubing straight was so painful. I gave chemotherapy to a paranoid schizophrenic who would wander off the ward barefoot when he had no white cells to fight infection. He received one medication in an intramuscular injection that I had to administer because the nurses were afraid he'd be violent. The oncologist supervising his care felt he deserved the prolonged, confining, painful, experimental treatment that he was totally unable to comprehend: I thought the oncologist was as crazy as the patient.

I almost quit my internship during the five weeks I spent on that ward. The oncologists would write the orders and go home to their families while we, the house staff, administered the drugs and watched the suffering. The straw that just about broke my back was the experimental hepatic artery line for chemotherapy. The idea was to deliver drugs directly to the liver to minimize systemic side effects and destroy tumor there. I don't keep up with the literature on the subject now, but as of the time I finished my residency there was no evidence that this gadget prolonged survival, although it did shrink livers enlarged with tumor. At the time we were sending patients to have the line placed and administering the drugs, there was almost no human data as to its efficacy.

One Sunday night, a retired college professor who was

entirely asymptomatic, had already outlived his six-month prognosis, and had just returned from a Mediterranean cruise was admitted for this procedure. He had been warned of possible side effects, but the principal investigator who had explained the procedure to him was entirely enthusiastic. In my few weeks on the service I had already seen how sick people could become from the drugs, and I felt that this man had been painted an overly optimistic picture. I pressed him to make sure he understood what was involved, and he did, so far as any layman could. After I examined him and found that his liver was not enlarged (scans had revealed the tumor present), I called my resident, who called the attending physician to argue that it did not seem right to subject a patient who was doing so well to such an untested procedure. The chief could not be dissuaded.

The patient was supposed to be in and out within the week. A month later, after he had survived a life-threatening infection and a blood clot in his leg, both clear complications of the therapy, he finally asked me, "You didn't really want me to have that line, did you?"

"No," I said, avoiding his eye.

"They told me all these things could happen. But I never could have imagined this." He was crying behind his thick glasses, as he did every morning on rounds. He never complained, he never whimpered—just tears.

I rotated off the service before he left the hospital, but I understand he did leave. We only wasted two months of his already borrowed time. The surgeons say you can't make a well man better, but we internists are bound and determined to try. No, my patient was not well, with a liver full of tumor, but he felt well, which should have counted for more than it did. "Life is a chess game," the chief told my resident over the phone. Sure, for him. My patient and I were the pawns.

On the cancer ward, I learned that I could pronounce three patients dead in one night, speak with each family, and roll right back to sleep. I learned that someone with half her face removed and with recurrent tumor raw at the surgical margins could joke about losing food out her cheek, and I could laugh. I learned too that it took tremendous emotional strength to interact with dying patients day after day, even more to humanely experiment with them, and that I did not have it. In fact, I didn't have the detachment or the stomach for academic medicine at all. Those five weeks of depressed exhaustion were as close to hell as I ever want to come. Only a supportive resident and a witty, sensitive fellow intern dragged me through.

After the bizarre rotations where I slogged along alone, the staff service seemed like easy street. My resident, who took call with me at night, was always at my elbow to direct me, and I was fortunate to land with pleasant colleagues. The pace was slower most of the time, more contemplative, and I had hit my stride. After a week's vacation in January, I realized that I was becoming a pretty good intern, efficient and diligent. Most of the patients were indistinguishable, though, even at the time. Unlike my student days, I was too busy to get to know many of them cordially and they were not silhouetted by the horror of the cancer unit. The scut list ruled my life, not the patients. On ward rounds, we interns grew impatient with the resident's teaching as we planned our day. In attending rounds, we revised our lists when we weren't catnapping after a night on call. We hoped for a beep so that we could leave without embarrassment: If the attending was boring or the students' presentations insufferable, we beeped each other out. We couldn't afford to attend teaching conferences because that represented an hour away from the ward. I ate bites of my lunch between phone calls to the lab or consultants. The afternoon was a mad scramble to stabilize everyone enough to sign them out to the covering intern without loose ends. In accordance with my shut-out-the-world policy, I never aimed for a specific departure time, but by never stopping, I usually managed to leave by six or seven on my nights off call. Since rounds started at eight and I had to pre-round in order to be sure I knew what had happened to my patients overnight, it was still a good twelve-hour day most of the time. Despite support hose and sensible shoes, my feet were always aching. In desperation, I even went to a podiatrist once, but his initial fee was $100, so I never went back.

We tended to rotate in small groups, so there were some interns I barely knew by name and one intern with whom I spent seven months. By mid-year, that intern and I worked together smoothly. Our goal was to allow the person who was not on call to leave as early as possible. Most compulsive medical interns function autonomously and are quite possessive about their patients: They stay until every test is done, until every result charted. My friend, who is now a surgeon, had a more pragmatic approach. "Look, I'm going to be here all night," he'd say. "I'll start the i.v. You go home." At first I was reluctant to let him, since the first rule of house-staff etiquette is never to pawn off your work on someone else. Of course, there were interns who would hear that a patient had a fever and walk out the door, signing the patient out as stable, but they were the lowest of the low. I didn't want anyone to consider me lazy. My friend would tease me, "You don't trust me with your patients, huh? You don't think I can handle them?" Since he is one of the smartest men I know, competent, dependable, and a down-home nice guy, I could hardly agree. So he would save me a little time wherever he could. I reciprocated on his days off, using the same line if he hesitated to leave. Aside from the time we saved each other, our rapport eased the pressure. The system worked because we respected each other and shared a similar medical philosophy. I did have misgivings about turning my patients over to some of my other colleagues. Rarely did I question their skill, but perhaps they had an abrasive manner or were too slow to intervene. Nevertheless, I would leave, unlike some guys who never went home. I was never the first out of the hospital but I was rarely the last either.

Leaving the hospital is a big deal. I once heard a pediatric chief resident praised for spending three days straight at the bedside of a critically ill child. The child had a one-to-one nurse, an intern, and a resident. Why did she need a guy who hadn't seen home in three days? She needed someone rested, with perspective, to be available to advise and supervise if needed. I suppose he lived alone and had nothing better to do. Or maybe he didn't trust the resident. I still don't see that as a model to emulate. Study after study of the effects of sleep deprivation back me up. After a while, you just have to let go.

So much of my energy internship year was devoted to pressing on, to making it day by day. I learned more than I ever have before or since, solely from experience. Interns aren't supposed to have time to read. Just as total-immersion language technique prepares the student to speak a foreign language quickly, so an internship prepares a doctor to act. While the fluent speaker may be good enough for government work, without a knowledge of the literature and culture that nourishes the language, his comprehension remains superficial. Certainly he can learn it later. And that's what residency is for, to learn about what you did as an intern. The danger is that internship may provide a false sense of competency that, together with sheer fatigue, smothers curiosity.

Lay people tend to view internship as a hazing experience without redeeming social value. That's not entirely true: Some of the stress and fatigue is necessary to develop the stamina required for practice. Interns also serve to staff hospitals at an hourly salary that works out to less than minimum wage. Society could not afford to pay a non-obligated physician to provide the around-the-clock emergency coverage it demands. So the taste that lingers from internship is exploitation. I think that exploitation was symbolized by our legal status. Before the National Labor Relations Board, we were students, with no right to collective bargaining. The university was not required to pay into Social Security. Yet before the Internal Revenue Service we were employees, taxed like anyone else.

Toward the end of the year, we started to dread promotion to new incompetency. We were good interns, but we did not feel ready for residency. I remember the night I knew I could take the next step. I was on call with my buddy, who had figured out that if we stuck with the traditional distribution of patients, taking every other admission, neither one of us would sleep. So we modified the order of admissions. Whichever person was up first would take two hits in a row while the other one slept "prophylactically." Then his work finished, the first intern would sleep while the second took the next two patients. Obviously, if only two patients were admitted, the second intern did no work. We both felt it was a gamble worth taking, however.

On the night in question, I was first up and had put my first patient to bed. It was close to midnight when a woman vomiting blood was admitted. I called my resident, who was asleep, to notify him and went down to the emergency room to pick her up. We arranged for an intensive care unit bed and I wheeled her out. The fellow on call in the intensive care unit was a pediatrician, ill at ease with this common adult problem. Since the patient was shocky from loss of fluid, I knew she needed a central intravenous line, which he had little experience starting. "Not to worry," I told him and started an i.v. in her right jugular vein, over her protests. She didn't want "no nurse sticking her." From the emergency room, I had called the gastroenterology fellow on call at home and presented the case. By the time I had stabilized the patient with fluid and transfusions, he had arrived to look into her stomach with a gastroscope for the source of bleeding. Surveying the name tags, mine and the pediatric fellow's, he immediately asked where my resident was. I hadn't missed him until then, but I realized he must have gone back to sleep. "I'll call him again if you like," I offered, "but I hate to wake him if we don't really need him." After all, I had him to supervise me. He agreed, although it was not standard operating procedure. It turned out that she was bleeding from dilated veins in the esophagus from liver disease caused by alcoholism. We gave her a drug that constricts blood vessels and eventually the bleeding slowed. The transfusions caught up with her loss and her blood pressure normalized.

Just after dawn, I was finishing my notes when I heard an invitation to breakfast. My partner, who had slept all night, was leaning over the desk, looking sheepish. I hadn't touched head to pillow, but I felt exhilarated. We rousted our resident, teasing him for sleeping through such an acute case, and headed down to chow. Even at the time, I realized that there were few cases of such a critical nature that I would have felt confident to handle myself. I had just seen enough bleeders to go on automatic pilot. Nevertheless, it was a great feeling to anticipate my new name tag, Medical Resident II.

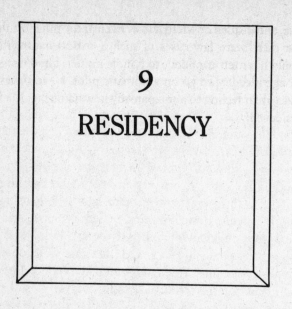

9
RESIDENCY

The difference between an intern and a resident can be summed up in one word: responsibility. This was symbolized in my program by a daily meeting called Resident's Report. At this conference, we discussed all the admissions from the previous twenty-four hours and criticized their management. A junior faculty member with major teaching responsibility led the analysis. Sometimes the chief of medicine or other faculty attended as well. Interns were not invited. I approached the report with mixed feelings. If I was rested and had not admitted the night before, it was a pleasant intellectual diversion to consider cases other than my own. If I had been up all night and was presenting complicated patients, it was a minor ordeal just to stay awake enough to keep the patients straight and respond to questions. I particularly enjoyed finding out what a smart group my fellow residents were. Their comments meant more to me than those of the faculty, who were not on the front line themselves and, as far as I was concerned, had all day to sit around and read.

I attended my first Resident's Report at the county hospital, where I started on the wards. The new interns had been on the ward a week when we arrived, just long enough to find the cafeteria. My first team consisted of two interns, one fourth-year student, and two third-year students. To my dismay, three of my five charges had entered medical school in my class. There was an intern who had taken a year off, a third-year student who had been held up by minor academic difficulties and maternity leave, and the fourth-year student had flunked two years. Faced with this group that I knew all too well, I immediately requested a change in personnel. It was trial enough to make the transition from intern to resident without trying to supervise students who were strictly my peers, not to mention friends. My petition was denied, for no apparent reason other than studied inflexibility. Since there were four medical teams, two headed by residents from other schools, it would have been simple to exchange a student or two.

This incident stuck in my craw, not because the consequences were disastrous—although the fourth-year student disappeared for a week and ultimately flunked the clerkship—but because it marked another loss of innocence. As an intern, I had to a large extent believed the party line that it was rough all over, that everyone simply had to grin and bear the schedule, the hours. As a resident, I quickly learned that the way the system actually worked was that those who worked hard were asked to work harder. No effort was made to try to ease life when possible, even when, as in the situation above, trouble lurked dead ahead, not around the corner.

The indifference to our plight was pervasive, but the one example that raises my ire to this day involved an overworked intern I encountered in the elevator. She was crying because she had already received eight admissions, and it was only noon of her twenty-four-hour admitting day. I had worked with her when she was a student, so I knew she was as capable as they come. I also knew that eight admissions to one intern before noon was extraordinary. It turned out that she was paired with an intern who had suffered a psychotic break, which had forced the staff to act. In order to ease his traumatic return to the wards after a period of intensive psychotherapy, she was getting 90 percent of the patients rather than half. Now, it was certainly necessary to coddle the disturbed intern. But the person who picked up the slack should not have been the other intern but the resident. A merciful resident would have admitted a few patients alone rather than kill the strong intern. Yet in the hierarchy of medicine, few doctors are big enough to stoop to work of the year behind. Furious at her exploitation, I stormed into the chief resident's office and warned him that he was breaking a good doctor by allowing the resident to admit so unevenly. He claimed ignorance and promised to speak to the resident. Perhaps he did. But that intern left the program at the end of the year, and the intern she was working overtime to protect— a weak, marginally competent doctor—stayed.

It is fair to say that I found supervising my various teams as taxing as treating the patients. I probably took the job too seriously, for one thing, and I had no teaching experience. Until residency, I had worked on the principle that if you want something done right, do it yourself. It was physically impossible to perform every task as a resident, however, and those residents who tried cheated their charges of the learning experience. I agonized over how much to let the interns have their own heads, whether to allow tardiness on rounds, what were reasonable expectations of the students. Sometimes it was easy to decide what to do. I remember a night of many admissions early in the year when my interns were flagging. About four A.M., the resident in the emergency room sent us a nearly comatose patient suffering kidney failure, who had several dangerous metabolic abnormalities and high blood pressure out of control. The intern next in line for an admission was an obstetrics intern fulfilling her medicine requirement. She was bright and well meaning, but her acute-care experience was shallow. Sure enough, faced with the patient in the intensive care unit, she sort of milled around, accomplishing nothing. Finally, I sent her to the lab to review slides of the patient's sputum so that we could determine if he had pneumonia. I set about what should have been her work, drawing blood and making sure the orders we had written were set in motion. About a half hour later, I realized that she had not returned from the lab, which was across the hall. I paged her, and she answered, flustered, "I'm so sorry. I fell asleep over the microscope."

My second month on the county wards, through a quirk of scheduling, I found myself heading an all-woman team. That was a delight. We worked well together and the stares as we swept through the halls were priceless. One pleasantly demented alcoholic used to entertain us every morning with diatribes against women in public office. He maintained that there were certain jobs that women simply could not perform. When we pointed out that every single one of his doctors was female, he would harrumph into his beard and bite his tongue until the next day. The admitting residents in the emergency room called us the girls, as in, "This is a tough case. Send in the girls." We suspected that they admitted every patient covered with lice to us out of turn; our team certainly specialized in critter removal. It only lasted a month, but it was fun.

The most stressful rotation of the residency, bar none, was my next month: emergency room at the county hospital. Now, instead of following orders, I had to give them. My assessment determined whether the patients were admitted and often whether they lived or died. There were supervisory physicians who floated through, but their specialty was second-guessing. They never seemed to be around in the crunch. Some of them were no help anyway. I must admit that it crossed my cynical mind to wonder why, if they were so smart, they chose to work for peanuts in that cesspool of humanity. Undoubtably altruism alone.

To keep people moving, you had to juggle many cases at once and be fierce about admissions and discharges. Some residents wanted to make the diagnosis in the emergency room and would hold patients, waiting for laboratory tests. I learned early on that all I had to decide was, dead or alive, in or out. As soon as I was confident that we had resuscitated a cardiac arrest victim, he was admitted to the coronary care unit. If a patient came in vomiting, dehydrated, and absolutely unable to keep down even sips of water, it didn't matter to me whether it was a virus or a bowel obstruction; he would have to be admitted. If the surgeons wanted him, fine. If not, it was "Admit Medicine." Since I was admitting to my fellow residents upstairs, I had to have the strength of my own convictions. Unlike private practice, in which another body means more money, salaried house officers never want another patient. It's just more work and less sleep. Certain cases of paramount clinical interest are the exceptions to this rule, but for every "fascinoma" there are ten vomiting alcoholics. Certain residents make a career of intimidating the guy in the emergency room. "What do you mean he needs to come in? I manage patients vomiting blood in my clinic all the time." The only answer to that comment is, "Well, I'm glad I'm not in your clinic. He's coming in." When my husband and I admitted to each other, we never discussed the indications, to avoid homicide. He and another friend used to call me The Rock when I was the admitting resident, so I know I wasn't a total pushover. The ultimate putdown was to be judged a "sieve," but my motto was, Better safe than sorry.

On the other hand, when a third-year student told me that he was having trouble understanding an elderly Filipino gentleman who refused to give any relative's name, I decided to see if I could communicate rather than wait for a translator. I spoke loudly and slowly and, to the amazement of the student, soon ascertained that the man wanted admission because his son had bought him a new, uncomfortable mattress and he thought the beds in the hospital might be more to his liking. Showing no mercy, I embarrassed him by stating that we ran a hospital, not a hotel, and scared him by threatening to make him pay out of pocket for his emergency room visit unless he immediately gave us his son's number. The wide-eyed student took the number, and the patient was dressed and waiting when his son arrived fifteen minutes after the call.

The part about paying was a lie and the whole tough-broad stance an act, but it was a hell of a lot more effective than trying to reason with him. I learned fast that all patients believe that their illness, no matter how trivial, is not only the most important problem in the world but deserves the doctor's undivided, immediate attention. People with sore throats would be angry because they had to wait while cardiac arrest patients were seen. After a while, you resign yourself to the fact that explanations of the purpose of an emergency room are futile and simply ignore the anger.

I also made short shrift of patients who refused blood drawing or other essential tests. My speech went something like this: "You need to be treated for your bleeding stomach. Treatment involves drawing your blood and putting a tube down your nose. If you don't have treatment, you may die; I cannot predict what will happen. It doesn't matter to me whether you come into the hospital or not. The decision is up to you. I cannot keep you against your will. But if you decide to leave, I must ask you to sign a paper that you are leaving against medical advice, because I think you should be in the hospital." I refused to beg mentally competent patients to stay. And I wanted to dispel the common illusion that they were doing the doctors a favor by accepting admission. Ludicrous as it sounds, I think some patients had the idea that we needed a certain quota of people to experiment on. The sad truth was that we all wished there was somewhere else to send them.

The hardest part for me during that chaotic month was switching roles. One moment I would be cajoling a little old lady into a pelvic exam, the next I would be screaming at a punk teenager trying to roll his guerney over to his girl friend. Or I'd have to console the relatives of a cardiac arrest victim who didn't make it, after browbeating a prostitute to make her admit to shooting dope. Twelve hours of this one-woman show would leave my nerves stretched and fraying. Fortunately, I am a cheap drunk and a beer would allow me to crash until my next shift. I know why doctors become addicts, though. I would have taken anything I needed to sleep. With only twelve hours between shifts, you can't afford to stay awake fretting over the decisions of the night before. Those who enjoy the emergency room life praise the excitement, the regular hours, and the absence of call. As a woman, I disliked having to prove I was really a doctor to a new face every ten minutes. In the emergency room, there is no opportunity to forge an ongoing doctor-patient relationship; saving lives is strictly doctor active, patient passive.

We all made mistakes. The most spectacular one our year occurred when a resident stopped the resuscitation effort on a young woman who had overdosed. She had arrived dead and after forty minutes of work remained without pulse, blood pressure, or respiration. The resident left the room to inform the family. He started talking to them in the waiting room, but a nurse interrupted and pulled him aside. "I think I saw her take a breath," she whispered. They started again, shocked her a couple of times, and her heart started beating in a regular rhythm. She lived almost a week in the intensive care unit. It turned out that her friends, finding her comatose, had tried to revive her by immersing her in a bathtub of ice water. Extreme hypothermia can mimic death because the body's functions are so slowed. Hence the maxim, You're never dead until you're warm and dead. Words to live by.

Another resident was called to evaluate a man with chest pain. The patient had known heart disease and frequent chest pain; he had been seen in cardiology clinic that day. There was nothing unusual about the duration or quality of the pain. In fact, the only reason he wound up in the emergency room was that he had been leaving the hospital when the pain occurred. Given this history and an unchanged cardiogram, my friend sent him home. He died later that night. Describing the incident and his otherwise slow day, my friend noted ruefully, "No hits, no runs, one error."

During our residency, we also did time in the emergency room of the university hospital. That was more a mom-and-pop operation, with none of the drama of the trauma center. There was plenty of time to shoot the breeze with the nurses and security guards. Every once in a while, one of the neighborhood schizophrenics would wander in to keep us on our toes. One gentleman a friend saw used to visit the emergency room once a year to ensure that the radio transmitter he claimed was in his head was still functioning. My friend checked the old chart and noted that the doctors had ordered skull X rays in years past, looking for a metal plate. Of course, the X rays showed nothing, but the patient wanted them again. In the interests of cost conservation, the resident took off his beeper and solemnly buzzed it around the patient's head a few times. He reported that the transmitter was working well and the patient left reassured.

Back on the wards, the major problem as the year progressed was contagious depression among the interns. Most of the time, I drew interns from other specialties who were just putting in their month of medicine. I supervised psychiatrists, anesthesiologists, radiologists, rotaters, and ob-gyn interns. In my more paranoid moments, I suspected they didn't trust me to teach a medical intern. The other residents pitied me, since nonmedical interns were stereotyped as uninterested and dull, but I found them eager to learn, although somewhat overwhelmed. My worst interns were two medical ones who combined depression and arrogance. An arrogant intern is a clear and present danger to patients because he will not ask for help or take advice. One intern I worked with insisted that he be allowed to see patients in chronological order. Nurses would be trying to reach him because admission number three was having chest pain, and he would refuse to come evaluate him because he was still talking to stable patient number one. He resented it if I evaluated a patient first, but the nurses would call me when he didn't respond. He would even skip seeing patients entirely if he wanted to sleep. On rounds, we were continually at loggerheads because he did not trust my judgment and I had no faith in his. He once left the hospital to buy a sandwich after a resident told him to keep a special eye on a new admission. Some of our destructive interaction may have been because I was a female authority figure, but he had run-ins with male residents also. Working with a guy like that made me long for the uncomplicated days of internship. I knew he was bright and terminally depressed, but his behavior was unbelievable. As usual, although our difficulty surfaced within the first week (even the third-year student came to me and complained about his attitude), we remained locked in mutual disgust for two months. No other resident wanted to be saddled with him since it was so much extra work to smooth the feathers he ruffled and to catch his omissions. Under duress, my husband volunteered to take him (he was afraid I'd kill the guy), but I didn't think that was fair. I heard later that intern made a pretty good resident. I think internship was simply beneath him.

With more reasonable interns, I tried to be supportive and cheerful. I took the team concept seriously and was not above splitting the scut list if the interns were hassled. My husband and I would host potluck suppers at the end of rotations, and I tried to provide positive feedback when I could. My model was a resident I had known as a student, a veritable Pollyanna. She would bounce down to the emergency room at two A.M. to pick up the most unsavory character in the world and act pleased to meet him. I did not approach her vigor, partly because my own fog of depression was always too thick, but I did raise some eyebrows. "Why are you always smiling?" friends would ask. What the hell else was there to do, I wanted to say.

I only completely cracked once, early on, when I was still at the county. Up all night, I had suffered through an interrogation in Resident's Report by the world's most pompous chief resident, which left me breathing fire. My team hadn't finished rounds, I didn't feel that I was an effective teacher, all the patients were deathly ill—it was hopeless. I tried to watch the medical conference televised from the university, but I realized that I couldn't see the screen through my silent tears. Finally, I leaned over to a resident I had worked with and respected the year before and asked if I could speak with him a moment. I didn't know him well but I poured out my frustration to him, and he listened for most of an hour. He told me he had felt the same way, that he had never finished rounds at the county, that I was doing as well as could be expected. A week later the powers that be announced that they were easing the first-year residents' schedules slightly. For months I thought the resident I had spoken to had somehow interceded, but he later denied passing on my anguish. I guess things looked bad all over.

When I came through, the second year of residency at our institution was mostly elective time, although I understand that now the ward and elective time is more evenly split between the two years, as it is in many other programs. It was almost like being a fourth-year student again, choosing subspecialty rotations at the various hospitals. I took nephrology (kidneys), pulmonary medicine (lungs), hematology-oncology (blood and cancer), dermatology, rheumatology (arthritis and related diseases), and gastroenterology (the gut). I specifically avoided cardiology, since I had landed with two months of coronary care as a junior resident. The glory of these rotations was that there was no night call associated with them, although each of us still had to take call about once a week as the senior resident in the house—a sort of general do-gooder, helping out where needed. I felt so much like a normal person again that I bought a pair of contact lenses, convinced that I would be rested enough to use them. Three of my fellow residents (male) all had the same idea. We were quite a group, blinking down the wards.

By and large, the electives were a disappointment. I had hoped for some guided study time, to read the specialty journals I had never had a chance to cover and to follow complicated patients on the consultant service. What I hadn't counted on was another kind of hierarchy, that of the subspecialty doctors, in which I was low man once again. A typical day started with rounds, led by the first-year fellow in nephrology, let's say. We would visit the patients referred previously for consultation by the house staff and discuss the previous day's developments. We noted our recommendations in the chart and often discussed them in person with the ward team as well. Attending rounds were held every other day on most services, daily on the busier ones. The attending would review the new cases and sign the formal consultation, prepared by a student, by me, or by the fellow. Particularly at the beginning of the year, when the first-year fellow was as green as I was, the attending was the only voice of experience. His signature was also required for billing purposes. In the afternoon, we would see new consults requested that day and attend conferences in a subspecialty such as pulmonary radiology or gastroenterologic pathology. Each subspecialty had its own grand rounds, a major clinical conference of the week, often attended by private physicians in the community as well as those in the university. A few days a week we would staff the outpatient clinic as well. Obviously, there was not much time for reading.

When the attending was interested in teaching and there were sufficient patients on the service, this system worked. On several services, however, personality conflicts dominated the experience. On one two-month rotation, there were two first-year fellows who disagreed on every point of patient management. They would bicker all through rounds. If he said blue, she said red. Then I was left to try to interpret their opposite recommendations to the ward team. On another service, it was the attendings themselves who argued through every conference. Yet another month, I rounded with a senior fellow who felt he was as qualified as the attending to direct patient management because of his additional training in a related field. Both of them apologized to me for the other's ruining my experience.

Finally, there was the service at which we would present the same patient over and over again at various conferences. I once heard the same case discussed three times in one day. It was not an esoteric problem and each attending had the same thoughts. Sitting on my hands to keep from fidgeting, I wondered whether the chief who organized our day in this manner believed that the ritual of the presentation was an end in itself, rather than learning about the patient's problem. I would find myself asking at the end of a particularly obscure discussion, "So what do you recommend that we tell the house staff?" I hope that my experience was merely rotten luck, rather than a reflection of the typical subspecialty approach to clinical dilemmas. Yet it was distressing to see how many times our suggestions offered little more than undirected speculation, and how the experts flatly contradicted each other.

The major new responsibility of my second and last year of residency was holding the Code Blue beeper, the one that announced cardiac arrests. The senior medical resident responded to every cardiac arrest and directed the subsequent resuscitation. Just picking up the beeper from the resident who held it for the previous twenty-four hours would raise my blood pressure. I jumped whenever a beeper went off. Since I carried my own beeper as a resident and might hold another while someone was in clinic, I did a lot of jumping. At night, I would bolt up every few hours to make sure the Code beeper was still working. Yet even a Nervous Nellie like me recognized the machismo of carrying three beepers on my belt. There was even an unspoken analogy between beepers and guns that surfaced during games of quick draw among the house staff.

When the Code Blue call came, I was supposed to run to the ward indicated. I joined the resuscitation team, which included an anesthesiologist and a surgeon. Typically, we'd be eating in the downstairs cafeteria when "Code Blue, twelfth floor" rang out. No time to wait for the elevator, so up eleven flights of stairs, whatever food we'd managed to eat weighing us down at every step. Once there, I was in charge of assessing the patient and directing the administration of drugs or electroshock to cajole the patient's heart into resuming a normal rhythm. The anesthesiologist took care of breathing for the patient and the surgeon cut if necessary. He might place a central intravenous line or even open the patient's chest.

Once I was actually running the Code, I stopped being

nervous. My mind switched into a mode that I recognized from the few times in my life I've been in physical danger. A very deliberate voice started talking out loud in a stream-of-consciousness evaluation, Lamaze for the panicked mind. "Okay, let's see, airway. Not breathing. Anesthesia here, placing tube. Okay. Chest compression. Pulse? Stop for a moment. No pulse. Electrocardiogram? (Louder) Cardiograph leads, please. We need an intravenous line, too. And a blood gas. Any history on this guy? When was his operation?" I would talk nonstop to myself, as though in a trance, just raising my voice for orders. I suspect people thought I was crazy, and in a sense I was. I certainly was not in my right mind. All I can say is that it worked. At least half of running a successful Code is keeping calm, establishing authority, and designating tasks. Most of the other half depends on the patient. Young healthy patients who are victims of a witnessed arrest tend to live. Old, chronically ill patients who were last seen three hours earlier don't do as well. There are standard algorithms for resuscitation, but the identity of the patient still matters. My trance was not deep enough to block out the general hysteria when the victim was very young or the arrest very unexpected. A mind reader would hear a chorus of "No, Lord, not this one."

Sometimes it worked, sometimes it didn't. "Calling," or ending, a Code was the final responsibility of the medical resident. If the patient had rigor mortis from the beginning it was easy to call it quits after a half hour or so. "That's it, ladies and gentlemen. Thanks for your help," the smooth residents would intone. If the patient was one who "should have made it," the effort would drag on for over an hour. Sooner or later, there comes a time when the patient's condition hasn't changed in quite a while and the effort fizzles. Everything that is within our power to correct has been corrected. No one has any new ideas except the surgeon, who suggests hopefully, "We could crack the chest?" That would be enough to jolt me out of my stupor. I would notice that my feet were hurting and that beneath all the tubing the patient was dead.

I cannot end a description of my training without devoting a few paragraphs to the institution that plagued us all more than any other during the three years of hospital medicine: general medicine clinic. Once a week, an afternoon was set aside for us to see outpatients, in order to give us some exposure to ambulatory medicine. We followed the same patients for three years, simulating a private practice as closely as possible. All hell could be breaking loose on the ward (and usually was, according to Murphy's Law), but at one o'clock we were due in clinic, our sacred, inviolable obligation. It took great strength of character to listen to a clinic patient complaining of constipation when someone on the ward was in extremis. Those of us who professed an interest in actually practicing medicine once we had served our time had to pretend that clinic was tolerable, although in fact I remember thinking more than once that if medicine in the real world was like clinic, I would have to retire before starting practice.

The problem was the patients. We saw chronically ill, indigent people who were unwanted elsewhere. In our overdoctored city, no one else escaped the clutches of private physicians. Some of these patients at one time cherished the illusion that they were receiving special care because they were "at the university," but after a few residents had come and gone, most of them abandoned that notion. They would roll in, crippled, blind, with charts of hospitalizations and laboratory tests several volumes thick. Faced with a stream of such patients with multiple medical problems, an average of five medications per patient, and often a language barrier as well, it took all of an intern's meager psychological reserves to gain control of the patient's therapy. My inclination was to admit everyone to the hospital, so at least I'd have a few days to read the charts. Only the joke of a senior resident kept me from the brink: "Just remember. If they were that sick, they'd be in the hospital."

So I made their acquaintance over weeks and months, finessing their care by simply renewing medications until I understood all their problems. From time to time, a patient would require admission, which was a traumatic experience, since it meant my peers would be reviewing my outpatient care. "We had to admit your clinic patient" was a call everyone dreaded. "What can you tell us about him?" Oh, God. No, I had not noticed the abnormal calcium value from three years ago. How to explain that half of each visit was wasted watching Mr. Jones, who was partially paralyzed and refused assistance, take off his jacket. And that he was so deaf I was never sure he heard what I was yelling at all. That I had never ordered volume two of his chart, which contained the abnormal calcium value, although the present volume was clearly marked, Volume four of four.

I grew attached to most of my clinic patients and they to me. When it came time for me to leave, they clucked their tongues and remembered the residents who had come before. I worried that some patients would suffer in the transition, since their problems were so complex and their therapy so delicate. One patient in particular, an eighty-year-old Vietnamese retired journalist, gave me pause. He had high blood pressure, kidney trouble, heart failure, and diabetes. We communicated in French, the second language of educated Vietnamese, but even that was difficult, since I realized a year into his care that the patient was mentally disturbed as well. From the beginning, he had insisted that his liver was the root of his problem. Once I had dissuaded him of that, I still often had trouble explaining his medications, which I attributed at first to my rusty French. He would go off on tangents, complaining about the political situation. Soon he started to send me thick envelopes full of newspaper clippings and paranoid ramblings (in French, of course) typed single-space—pages and pages about the decline of the United States due to homosexuals, or the young, or blacks. Despite my wedding ring, these missives were addressed to Mademoiselle La Doctoresse, care of medical clinic. The staff teased me about love letters from my patients. Monsieur expected me to read them for discussion at the next opportunity. He viewed his monthly visit as an informal tutorial in current affairs. I struggled to cut him off and talk medicine, but it still took me twice as long to see him as the schedule allowed.

His idol was Nelson Rockefeller, who had once responded to one of those letters. During one of our later visits, he proudly displayed the form letter he had received, bearing the then Vice President's signature. I didn't have the heart to comment on the circumstances of Rockefeller's death, but I know the incident upset him because he stopped talking about the great man.

In the last few months of my senior residency, I arranged for Monsieur to be followed by a Vietnamese house officer, even though it meant transferring him to another medical clinic. I discussed the transition with both of them and set the chart in order. One day shortly before the end, I received a call on the ward informing me that Monsieur had died in his sleep and asking if I would sign the death certificate. I was stunned, although I, of all people, knew his health was fragile. The timing was too coincidental. "He didn't want you to leave, Doctor," commented the receptionist in medical clinic.

At that point I was having second thoughts, too. For better or for worse, the teaching institution had been my home for the last seven years. Most of my friends, including my husband, were continuing or had plans to come back after a year. Perhaps doctors in the real world were actually avaricious bunglers, as they were portrayed in the university. Should I look for a salaried job or go into practice on my own? Did I want to work full-time? When should I think about having a child? Frankly, I was so tired of medicine I didn't feel like working at all.

Monsieur's death was a catalyst, releasing me from the past. My training was over and it was time to move on. Summoning all my courage, I let myself hope for the first time in seven years that next year would truly be better.

Epilogue

I remember the last day of internship because my team dressed up in three-piece suits, "like private docs." I can't remember the last day of residency. I didn't have a job or a fellowship lined up. I don't think I truly believed my training would ever end. If I imagined it at all, I thought the transition to practice would be dramatic, that I would magically acquire a wardrobe of tasteful suits and a heavy car. An aura of physicianhood would envelope me, repelling skeptical glances and nursing inquiries. Patients would respect me because of my background, not in spite of it.

It hasn't worked out quite that way. I am a member of a three-person private-practice group, but I am salaried, which sets me apart from most of my colleagues. In the doctor's lounge, which I visit solely for the free coffee, I can't participate in the conversations about investments and yachts. Only the nurses ask to see my baby pictures.

I feel at home now on the wards, but my social life still revolves around potluck suppers, not the opera.

After three months' unpaid maternity leave, I have returned to working about a forty-hour week. My contract expires in a few months, however, and will not be renewed. My boss has decided that he cannot afford to pay me a salary anymore because of the economic depression. So I have a choice of striking out on my own or finding another salaried job. Although I haven't weighed all the options yet, I am leaning toward the security and predictability of a large prepaid health plan. Time is my first priority, not money or autonomy. I am willing to work a full-time week, but not the sixty hours of the typical internist in private practice. It will be a relief to lay down the dual burdens of primary breadwinner and primary child-care provider when my husband finishes his fellowship this year. Entering our thirties, nine years after leaving college, we are both looking forward to charting our own course.

Index

Index

Index

Index

Index

Index